BOOK of JOOK

A Healthy Alternative to the Typical Western Breakfast

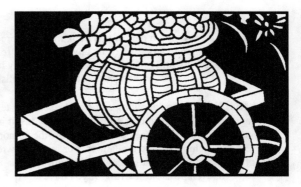

CHINESE MEDICINAL PORRIDGES

Bob Flaws

BLUE POPPY PRESS, INC

Published by:
BLUE POPPY PRESS, INC.
5441 Western Avenue #2
Boulder, CO 30301

First Edition, February, 1995
Second Printing, May, 1998
Third Printing,February, 2001

ISBN 0-936185-60-0 LC 94-77986
COPYERIGHT 2001 © BLUE POPPY PRESS

WARNING: When following some of the self-care techniques given in this book, failure to follow the author's instruction may result in side effects or negative reactions. Therefore, please be sure to follow the author's instructions carefully for all self-care techniques and modalities. For instance, wrong or excessive application of moxibustion may cause local burns with redness, inflammation, blistering, or even possible scarring. If you have any questions about doing these techniques safely and without unwanted side effects, please see a local professional practitioner for instruction.

DISCLAIMER: The information in this book is given in good faith. However, the author and the publishers cannot be held responsible for any error or omission. The publishers will not accept liabilities for any injuries or damages caused to the reader that may result from the reader's acting upon or using the content contained in this book.

COMP Designation: Original work and functionally translated compilation

Printed at Sheridan Books, Inc., Chelsea, MI on recycled paper
Interior design by Honora Lee Wolfe
Cover design by Eric J. Brearton
10 9 8 7 6 5 4

PREFACE

This book is about Chinese medicinal congees. It is intended for use by professional practitioners of Traditional Chinese Medicine and the patients under their care. I have written it in response to numerous questions by my patients and students about what to eat for breakfast. It is also part of my on-going efforts to establish healthier eating habits in the West in general. In my experience, diet is central to both the development and treatment of chronic, recalcitrant diseases. Medicinal congees are some of the healthiest meals a person can eat. They should not be overlooked by anyone interested in preventing or treating disease.

The formulas in this book have been compiled from a number of Chinese language sources. These include *Zhong Hua Shi Wu Liao Fa Da Quan (A Great Collection of Foodstuff Treatments in China)* published by the Jiangsu Science & Technology Press, *Yin Shi Liao Fa (Food & Drink Therapy)* published by the Guandong Technical Press, *Da Zhong Yao Shan (Medicinal Meals of the Masses)* published by the Sichuan Science & Technology Press, *Qian Jin Shi Zhi (Food Treatments [from the Prescriptions Worth a] Thousand [Pieces of] Gold)* and *Shi Liao Fang (Food Treatment Formulas)* both published by Commercial Press of China, *Pian Fang Da Quan (A Great Collection of Folk Formulas)* published by the Beijing Science & Technology Press, and *Zhong Guo Yao Shan (Medicinal Meals of China)* published by the Shanghai College of TCM Press.

Medicinal identifications are based on Bensky & Gamble's *Chinese Herbal Medicine: Materia Medica*; Hong-yen Hsu's *Oriental Materia Medica: A Concise Guide*; Stuart & Reid's *Chinese Materia Medica*; and *Zhong Yao Da Ci Dian (The Encyclopedia of Chinese Medicinals)* published by the Shanghai Science & Technology Press.

The translational terminology is based on Nigel Wiseman's *Glossary of Chinese Medical Terms and Acupuncture Points* published by Paradigm Publications, Brookline, MA.

Bob Flaws
August, 1994

CONTENTS

BOOK I

INTRODUCTORY THEORY

BOOK II

TREATMENT FORMULARY

CONTENTS

BOOK I

INTRODUCTORY THEORY

CHAPTER 1

THE PROBLEM WITH BREAKFAST

Sun Si-miao, the greatest Chinese doctor of the Tang Dynasty (618-907 ce), said that the superior doctor should first adjust the patient's diet and lifestyle. Only if that does not eliminate the patient's disease should the doctor go on to administer acupuncture or herbs. This statement shows how important dietary therapy is in Traditional Chinese Medicine or tcm. Without a healthy diet and lifestyle, acupuncture and Chinese herbal medicine alone cannot truly heal or prevent the recurrence of chronic disease. However, as a TCM practitioner in the West, whenever I explain to my patients the do's and don'ts of a healthy diet, the question inevitably arises, "But what do I eat for breakfast?"

For most Westerners, breakfast is the most problematic and unhealthy meal of the day. What do we typically eat? Either a) greasy, fatty, high cholesterol foods, such as eggs, sausage, bacon, ham, and butter; b) sweets and sugars, such as donuts, cakes, sweet rolls, jams, jellies, syrups, and sugar-coated cereals; c) chilled milk and milk products, such as cold milk on top of cereals and yogurt; or d) some combination of the above—all of which we wash down with orange juice and/or coffee.

We all know that excess dietary fat and cholesterol are bad for us, bad for our hearts and arteries and bad for our immune systems, and certainly not good for our waistlines. Most of us also know that sugar is bad for us as well. It can cause both hypoglycemia and hyperglyce-

3

mia (*i.e.*, diabetes). But it also stresses the adrenal glands and thus depresses the immune system at the same time as it prompts the body to produce more cholesterol as a stress response. In addition, the metabolism of sugar and sweets uses up great quantities of vitamins, minerals, and certain proteins as well. Thus, although sugar can make us overweight, it can also make us undernourished. One other thing that sugars and sweets do is to feed internal populations of yeast and fungi in the body. Such overgrowths of yeast and fungi are often generically referred to as candidiasis, and candidiasis is associated with allergies, autoimmune disorders, and the progression of many chronic diseases, including multiple sclerosis (MS), systemic lupus erythematosus (SLE), rheumatoid arthritis (RA), AIDS, cancer, chronic fatigue immune deficiency syndrome (CFIDS), and a long list of others.

It is also increasingly well known that many people do not digest milk and milk products well. Not only are whole milk products a source of fats and oil, but many people lack the enzymes to break milk down. Further, many people have food allergies to milk and milk products. Also, many people understand that milk is a mucus-forming food. Although drinking breast milk is essential for the health of the infant and toddler, drinking cold, pasteurized milk out of the refrigerator and eating diary products such as cheese and yogurt may not be all that healthy for adults.

Nonetheless, even Chinese medicine says that breakfast should be the most nutritious meal of the day. As the Chinese saying goes, "Eat a good (hearty) meal in the morning, enough food at noon, and not much in the evening." And aren't our typical Western breakfast foods highly nutritious? Yes, they are. But, according to Chinese medicine, that is their problem. They are, in a sense, too nutritious, and so they overload our system and gum up our internal works. In order to understand this fact, we must first understand something about how Chinese medicine views digestion and then about the Chinese medical descriptions of these foods.

4

CHAPTER 2

CHINESE MEDICINE
& DIGESTION

Chinese medical theory likens the process of digestion to the process of distillation in the making of alcohol. This process begins with the stomach. The stomach is likened to a large pot on a stove or a large fermentation vat. Foods and liquids enter the stomach where they are "rottened and ripened." In other words, they are turned into a 100°F soup or mash (38° C). Until they are turned into this 100° soup, no further digestion can take place.

The fire under this pot is the spleen, or at least Chinese medicine's concept of the spleen. It is the qi from the spleen which, like a fire under a still, transforms the mash, separating the pure essence from the dregs, and driving this pure essence upward. In Chinese medicine, the pure part of food and liquids distilled by the spleen and sent up to the heart and lungs to become the qi and blood is called the *jing wei* or finest essence, and the arising of this pure or clear qi is referred to as the upbearing of the clear. Then the stomach sends the impure of turbid dregs downward for excretion as urine and feces. This is referred to as the downbearing of the turbid.

Thus, in Chinese, digestion is referred to as *xiao hua*. *Hua* means to transform and stands for the transformation of the pure part of foods and liquids into qi and blood. *Xiao* means to disperse, and this stands for the dispersal of the turbid residue. The process of sending the clear upward and the turbid downward is called the qi mechanism. And the spleen and stomach together are also referred to as the *zhong jiao* or middle burner. They are the middle since they are found in the area between the bottom of the ribs and the belly button. They are a burner since their transformations are warm transformations similar to cooking. In Chinese, the character *jiao* or burner is written as a bird roasting over a fire and clearly implies the concept of cooking. Thus in a nutshell, we can say that digestion begins by turning all foods and liquids into 100° soup in the stomach, and, as a corollary of that, the closer a food is to 100° soup, the more easily digestible it is.

Following along this same metaphor, it is easy to understand why eating cold and raw foods make them less digestible. Cooking is a form of predigestion, and, since the process of digestion is a warm transformation, foods should be eaten at approximately body temperature for easiest and most complete digestion. In addition, foods should be well chewed or otherwise broken down so as to more easily "rotten and ripen." And further, there should be enough liquid in the stomach to make a soup but not enough to douse the fire of digestion.

*S*PLEEN *&* *S*TOMACH AS *P*OSTNATAL *R*OOT

Because the spleen and stomach are the first and pivotal organs in the creation of qi and blood from food and liquids consumed, they are referred to as the postnatal root of qi and blood production. The spleen and stomach are so important in human physiology according to Chinese medicine that Jin Zi-jiu, a late nineteenth century Chinese doctor wrote this about them:

> As the essence and mind of humankind look to earth as their abode, the ten thousand things look to earth as their root. When the postnatal spleen and stomach attain force, the righteous and original qi are able to fulfill themselves. Humankind's qi mechanism and yin and yang rest entirely upon the authority of the spleen and stomach. Humankind's heavenly righteous qi is all in the stomach. Therefore, nurturing the stomach's *jin* or fluids is the plain way to supplement vacuity.

> The stomach rules holding the food. The spleen governs transportation and transformation. The stomach is yang earth, while the spleen is yin earth. Stomach yang relies on spleen yin for moistening just as spleen yin borrows stomach yang for warming. The spleen and stomach serve as the

6

interior and exterior and are the spring of postnatal generation and transformation. By the one act of treating the spleen, three good results will come: First, flourishing spleen qi is like a blue sky on a wonderful day with dragons and lightning subdued from attack. Secondly, flourishing spleen qi allows essence and qi to roam overflowingly and supply upwards the lungs. And finally, flourishing spleen qi allows the pure essence of water and grain to replenish the blood before it reaches exhaustion.

The hundreds of diseases of the four seasons all originate in the stomach. As the stomach gets grain, improvement comes. Therefore, if the diet is improved one inch, the disease pathogen is forced back one inch. Consequently, in chronic diseases, sleep and diet must be emphasized. Sleeping unsettled and eating irregularly, how will the fluids and humors regenerate, and what will maintain the mechanisms of production? After illness, readjust the spleen and stomach. Relying on the middle qi to gain authority, dietary evils and repletions can transform and resolve themselves. Moreover, liver yang, qi, and fire will not be able to float upward.[1]

Further, explaining the qi mechanism, Jin Zi-jiu has this to say:

... counterflow means difficult respiration and chaos is turbulent upbearing and downbearing. When clear yang qi cannot filter through, then the flows of rising and falling stagnate and the distribution of fluids becomes erratic. Thus the clear that rises and the turbid that descends rely entirely on the middle venter's motion. Because the spleen and stomach reside in the middle, they are the real directors of inhaling and exhaling. With the middle venter wide open, the upbearing and downbearing of clear and turbid cannot be impeded. The bowels and portals flow freely and are open. Thus the rise and fall of the stomach and spleen dictate the whole body's qi mechanism. If the middle burner's foundation is not set in solid rock, then upbearing and downbearing are shifty, breathing is stuffy, and the qi that is grasped does not collect in the reservoirs. Thus the refined essence seeps out but is not spread properly. Wrong steps are taken in all directions, and yin and yang counterflow chaotically.[2]

---

[1] Jin Zi-jiu, *Jin Zi Jiu Zhuan Ji* (*A Collection of Jin Zi-Jiu's Special Understanding*), Peoples Health & Hygiene Press, Beijing, 1982, p. 66-7

[2] *Ibid.*, p. 68

From the above, it is clear that in Chinese medicine anything which benefits and promotes digestion promotes the health of the entire organism, while anything which impedes or hinders digestion can harm the health and well-being of the entire body. Thus is the pivotal and exalted role of the spleen and stomach and consequently diet in Chinese medicine.

CHINESE MEDICINE'S DESCRIPTIONS OF INDIVIDUAL FOODS

Just as every medicinal herb and substance has its own individualized Chinese medical description in TCM, so does every food. In other words, in TCM, each food has its own flavors, nature (meaning temperature), direction, channel entering (or the organs on which it exerts its greatest influence), functions, indications, and contraindications. If we know each of these various aspects about a food, we can, according to both TCM theory and 2,000 plus years of Chinese written and recorded clinical experience, know what effect that food will have on any given individual. In other words, if we know the patient's TCM pattern diagnosis, we can tell if any food will either benefit that person or make them sick (or sicker).

For instance, take the TCM description of rice. Rice's flavor is sweet and its nature or temperature is neutral. The directional effect it has on the qi of the body is upbearing. That means that rice tends to promote the arising of clear qi in the body. In terms of functions, rice fortifies the spleen and boosts the qi at the same time as it harmonizes the stomach. This means that rice significantly helps generate and transform qi at the same time as it promotes good digestion. In addition, rice quenches thirst, relieves mental depression, and stops diarrhea due to spleen vacuity. Therefore, rice is recommended in the TCM dietary treatment of indigestion, nausea, vomiting, diarrhea, and vexatious thirst due to summerheat.

Now let us look at pork. Pork's flavor is sweet and salty. Its nature or temperature is also neutral. Its direction is both upbearing and downbearing. Its functions are that it supplements the kidneys, enriches yin, and moistens dryness. Therefore, pork is used to treat kidney vacuity low back pain, spermatorrhea, night sweats, and senile deafness, all believed to be symptoms of kidney yin vacuity according to Traditional Chinese Medicine.

QI & WEI

If we compare the medicinal or physiological effects of rice and pork, we see that rice's effect is primarily to boost the qi, while pork's effect is primarily to nourish yin. This dichotomy underscores a basic dichotomy among all foods. Comparatively, rice has more qi and pork has more *wei*. *Wei* means flavor, but when talking about foods and Chinese medicinals, *wei* implies something which is dense, moist or bloody, slightly greasy or slippery, and which can enrich and nourish yin substance. As such, foods high in flavor or *wei* are highly nutritious but also tend to be hard to digest and can overstuff the qi mechanism, thus disrupting upbearing of the clear and downbearing of the turbid.

We need both qi and *wei* in our diet, but for good digestion and therefore good health, we should eat relatively more foods high in qi and less high in *wei*. Most of the foods eaten as part of the typical Western breakfast are high in *wei*. This includes all the meats, milk, yogurt, cheese, and eggs. As mentioned above, foods high in *wei* tend to be dense and moist. This means that they can easily cause a pathological accumulation of dampness and phlegm.

SUGAR & SWEETS

According to Chinese medicine, the sweet flavor enters the spleen. In small, naturally occurring amounts, as in most grains, meats, and many vegetables like carrots, squash, peas and beans, the sweet flavor helps to fortify the spleen and supplement the qi. But the sweet flavor also generates body fluids. In Chinese philosophy based on the *Yi Jing* or *Classic of Change*, there is the idea that anything when it reaches its extreme will tend to transform into its polar opposite. In the case of sugar and sweets, when very concentrated or in large amounts, they still enter the spleen but, instead of making the spleen stronger, they make it weaker. In this case, the dampness associated with the sweet flavor overwhelms and impedes the spleen's function. Thus evil dampness accumulates and gums up the works. This spleen weakness and dampness may then manifest as fatigue, bodily weakness and heaviness, edema, and all sorts of digestive complaints, including loss of appetite, nausea, vomiting, abdominal distention, and diarrhea.

As mentioned above, one of the elements of the typical Western breakfast is a tendency toward sweets and sugars. Orange juice and other fruits and juices are all very sweet and dampening. Sugar, honey, molasses, maple syrup, glazes and fillings, jams and jellies are all likewise sweet and dampening. At first, eating sugar or something sweet gives one an immediate boost of energy. However, after a little bit, instead of feeling energized, we typically feel fatigued. This is when we Westerners go on coffee break and have some caffeine and more sugar to try to boost us up again. Unfortunately, this is merely a quick fix and only perpetuates the problem it attempts to remedy.

WHEAT

In the West, bread is considered the staff of life, and by this we typically mean wheat bread and other risen and baked products. However, just as rice has its own Chinese medical description, so does wheat. According to TCM, wheat is sweet in flavor but cool in nature. It enters the spleen, heart, and kidneys. Its qi is downbearing, while its functions are to clear heat and downbear yang, nourish the heart and calm the spirit, supplement the kidneys and quench thirst. In addition, wheat is used in TCM to treat insomnia, vexation and agitation, spontaneous sweating, night sweats, dry mouth and throat, and menopausal complaints.

When a Chinese doctor reads this description, he or she immediately knows that, compared to rice, wheat has more *wei*, that it is more difficult to digest, and that it tends to be dampening. These negative aspects of wheat are magnified when the wheat is eaten as refined flour in the form of bread or pasta. Li Dong-yuan, one of the four great masters of internal medicine of the Jin-Yuan Dynasties (1280-1368 CE) and author of the *Pi Wei Lun (Treatise on the Spleen & Stomach)*, repeats over and over again that a person with weak spleen function and a tendency to dampness should not eat "steamed wheat buns" or dumplings. Although our white bread and refined flour products are made differently than steamed wheaten buns, nevertheless, they have the same effect on digestion. This includes most of the breads, rolls, croissants, and other baked goods we tend to consume at breakfast.

YIN FIRE

Obviously the man who wrote *Treatise on the Spleen & Stomach* had a lot to say about the spleen, diet, and dampness. In fact, Li Dong-yuan is the Chinese doctor who raised the spleen and stomach to the pivotal and important role described by Jin Zi-jiu more than six centuries later. However, Li did not content himself with saying that a weak spleen causes indigestion. Rather, he laid out a careful but complicated scenario of how a weak spleen or anything that weakens the spleen can cause all sorts of complicated, obstinate, chronic diseases.

Let's say the spleen has become weak due to faulty diet, overfatigue, excessive worry, or lack of exercise. In that case, the spleen, which is one of the main viscera involved in water metabolism, may not transport and transform body fluids correctly. These fluids may then accumulate and transform into evil or pathological dampness. Dampness, because it is heavy tends to percolate downward from the middle burner to the lower burner. The lower burner is the lower abdomen. Because dampness is yin, it obstructs the free flow of yang qi. Because qi is yang, it is warm. As this warm qi backs up behind this accumulating dampness, the warmth of the qi may and commonly does transfer this heat to the evil dampness which then becomes damp heat.

Damp heat in the lower burner can cause a number of pathological conditions. In the bladder and urinary tract, it can cause cystitis, prostatitis, and kidney stones. In the intestines, it can cause hemor-rhoids, diarrhea, hemafecia, ulcerative colitis, and rectal prolapse. In a woman's reproductive organs, it can cause pelvic inflammatory disease, endometriosis, infertility, and vaginal tract infections. In a man's reproductive organs, damp heat can cause spermatorrhea and infertility. In both men and women, it may be associated with herpes genitalia.

However, damp heat in the lower burner may also injure the liver and kidneys. According to Li, damp heat injuring the liver and kidneys results in atony of the lower limbs. In modern terms, Li was talking about such paralytic and progressive atrophic, autoimmune diseases as MS and SLE. In terms of the kidneys alone, damp heat injures their source of transformation. In that case, kidney yang loses its root in the lower burner or abdomen and tends to float upward where it further damages the spleen and stomach and collects in the heart and lungs. When this heat accumulates in the heart, it manifests as men-tal/emotional problems. When it accumulates in the lungs, it manifests as respiratory problems, such as asthma and allergies, and as skin diseases, such as acne, eczema, and psoriasis. Because the yang qi of the kidneys flushes upward, the lower body is left cold, but the upper body tends to become too hot and inflamed.

This upward heat associated with damp heat below was named yin fire by Li Dong-yuan. It is yin because of the dampness but fire because of the heat. It causes chaos in the upbearing and downbearing of the clear and turbid qi of the entire body and eventually affects all the organs and bowels of the entire organism. It is this scenario that best describes most of the chronic, recalcitrant, and often even life-threatening diseases which seem so prevalent in modern Western society. These include MS, SE, RA, AIDS, CFIDS—a.k.a. myalgic encephalopathy or ME in the UK and Europe, diabetes mellitus, chronic sinusitis, multiple allergies, polysystemic chronic candidiasis, endometriosis, autoim-mune thyroiditis, autoimmune ovaritis and infertility, and the Big C, cancer.

As a TCM clinician treating Western patients, over and over again I see chronic conditions affecting the spleen and stomach, liver and kidneys, heart and lungs, intestines, bladder, and reproductive systems with heat above and cold below, and dryness above due to that heat and damp heat below at the same time as there is coldness. This is exactly what Li Dong-yuan was writing about at the time of Genghis Khan, and these are exactly the kinds of diseases in which the spleen and stomach are pivotal. In addition, they are also the kinds of conditions that are inextricably tied to diet, for better and for worse.

I am not saying that all these diseases are due solely to improper diet, but, in my experience, in all cases of yin fire associated with spleen vacuity weakness, improper diet is *the single most important factor* in such diseases' worsening. Conversely, a proper diet is the cornerstone in such diseases' remedial treatment. Without such a proper diet, it is difficult if not impossible for acupuncture and Chinese herbal medicine to achieve either satisfactory or lasting results. As we have seen above, the typical Western breakfast is a recipe for spleen vacuity and dampness which then may transform into damp heat.

CHAPTER 3

THE QING DAN DIET

So now you are saying, "If I don't eat eggs, bacon, cheese, milk, yogurt, toast and jam, sweet rolls or Danish pastry or drink orange juice, then what can I eat for breakfast?" Aye, there's the rub. The general answer is a *qing dan* diet. *Qing* means clear or pure but it also means light. *Dan* means bland. Bland foods tend to be the opposite of foods high in *wei* or flavor. This is the diet that Chinese medicine believes is the foundation of good health and long life.

A *qing dan* diet is a diet composed mainly of grains, beans and bean products, vegetables, and fruits. Such a diet is low in animal protein such as meat, eggs, milk, and fish. When these are eaten, they are eaten only sparingly and not every day. Such a diet is also low in sugars and sweats and fats and oils. Grains, beans, vegetables, and fruits are all foods which are relatively high in qi as opposed to *wei*. They therefore promote the arising of clear yang or the pure qi and are the opposite of foods which are heavy in turbid, dense, and dampening *wei* or flavor. Thus grains, beans, vegetables, and fruits are relatively *qing* or pure and light compared to animal proteins, fats, and oils being turbid or *zhuo*.

A *dan* or bland diet also refers to one that is low in spicy, peppery foods, fermented foods, such as soy sauce, vinegary foods, salt, and alcohol. These foods also tend to cause or aggravate damp heat. Zhu Dan-xi, a disciple of a disciple of Li Dong-yuan and himself another of the four great masters of medicine of the Jin-Yuan Dynasties, explains the benefits of eating a *qing dan* diet in a chapter of his *Ge Zhi Yu Lun* (*Extra Treatises Based on Investigation & Inquiry*):

Some may ask, "The *Nei Jing* states that insufficient essence should be supplemented with *wei*. It is also stated that the earth feeds human beings with the five flavors or *wei*. The ancients began to eat meat at the age of 50, but your honor, now as old as 70, (even yet) abstains completely from salt and vinegar. Have you acquired the *dao* (*i.e.*, become a saint)? (If not,) how does your honor manage to keep your spirit thriving and your complexion shining?"

The answer is that some of the flavors are a gift from heaven and others are produced by human endeavor. The gifts from heaven include, for instance, grains, beans, greens, and fruits which are moderate and harmonious flavors. When eaten as food by humans, these result in supplementing yin. These are what are referred to in the *Nei Jing* (*The Inner Classic*).

Those which human endeavor produces are the thickish flavors made by means of brewing and blending in the process of cooking. These carry toxins that cause illness and fell life. It is these sort of flavors that you are suspicious of. Abstention from salt and vinegar is not truly eating bland. The saltiness in barley and chestnut, the sweetness in rice and yam, and the acridity in scallion and garlic, these are all flavors (too). Do you consider them bland?

The hearts of those who rest content with moderate and harmonious flavors are restrained and fire (in them) is downborne. Those who are happy (only) with thickish flavors indulge (*i.e.*, let loose) overwhelming fire. There is no doubt (about this). The *Nei Jing* also states, "That which is generated by yin is rooted in the five flavors." These are certainly the flavors bestowed by heaven. And that which damages the five palaces of yin (*i.e.*, the five viscera) are (also) the five flavors. (But) these are certainly the flavors produced by human endeavor. Thus the teaching of the sage (*i.e.*, the Yellow Emperor) for the protection of the people is all-embracing.[3]

In the above passage, Zhu Dan-xi explicitly says that one does not need to eat a diet rich in thick, heavy foods and flavors in order to get plenty of nourishment. According to Chinese medical theory, if one eats a diet of mostly grains, beans, vegetables, and fruits, chews well, and digests their food well, as long as they get adequate exercise but do not overtax

---

[3] Zhu Dan Xi, *Ge Zhi Yu Lun* (*Extra Treatises Based on Investigation and Inquiry*), trans. by Yang Shou Zhong and Duan Wu-jin, Blue Poppy Press, Boulder, CO, 1994, p. 117-8

their body and qi, whatever qi and blood that is made but not used each day will be converted into yin essence at night during sleep. This yin essence nourishes and strengthens the physical body and its substance. Thus, even though foods such as grains and vegetables may not be full of yin-nourishing *wei*, their qi will be transformed into yin as long as one's digestion, rest, and exercise are harmonious.

When I was a student at the Shanghai College of Traditional Chinese Medicine, I once had a conversation with my teachers about this issue of nourishing yin and enriching essence through dietary means. They mentioned that outside hospitals in China where a lot of cancer patients are treated there are always several people selling turtles. Turtle meat is believed to be a very powerful yin supplement. As a food it is very high in *wei*. Advanced cancer patients typically exhibit symptoms of yin vacuity and, therefore, eating turtle seems like the perfect remedy. However, my teachers pointed out that cancer patients typically also have weak spleens and even turbid dampness or damp heat. Turtle meat is hard to digest, easily damages the spleen, and further gums up the qi mechanism. Therefore, although in theory turtle meat should be good for those suffering from yin vacuity, in actual practice, the safer method of nourishing yin and filling essence is to eat a *qing dan* diet which is easily and completely digestible.

THE QING DAN DIET IN THE WEST

The *qing dan* diet of Traditional Chinese Medicine is essentially the diet currently recommended by the United States Department of Agriculture which has switched from promoting the so-called four food groups to the "Eating Right Pyramid." This pyramid shows that the basis for a healthy diet should be whole grains and complex carbohydrates. These should then be followed in amount by vegetables and fruits. Next, one should eat some animal protein and dairy products but at a much lesser amount. And finally, one should only use very sparingly sweets, salts, fats, and oils. The *qing dan* diet is also essentially the same as the Pritikin Diet and the Macrobiotic Diet.

The *qing dan* diet has always been the traditional diet of most poor people throughout the world living in temperate regions. It is only in the last 100 years in the West that poor and middle class people have been able to indulge themselves with meat, sugar, fruit juices, fats and oils. In Chinese medicine, it is a long-held belief that peasants are healthier than rich people because of their hard work and simple diet. As Zhu Dan-xi says in his *Ge Zhi Yu Lun*, "Those poor and humble people in the mountains and wilderness know nothing but a bland and homely (diet), but their movements never betray decrepitude and their bodies remain safe and sound (their entire lives)."[4]

This belief has recently been corroborated by a large scale study conducted in China jointly by Oxford University, Cornell University, and the Chinese Academy of Preventive Medicine in Beijing. This study is the largest ever undertaken of a nation's eating habits and health consequences. For two years, the subjects, aged 34-64, were interviewed about their eating and other habits, such as smoking and drinking. Blood samples were taken to measure cholesterol and other such things. Dietary records were obtained and the foods consumed were weighed and measured. Among the important findings were the facts that:

1. Chinese consume many more vegetables, grains, and fruits than Americans and Britons.

2. The daily fiber intake of the average Chinese is 3 times more than the average American.

3. The average Chinese derives anywhere from 6-24% of their daily calories from fat, compared to 39% for the average American and 45% for the average Briton.

4. In most of the counties included in this study, people eat meat only about once per week. In countries where meat is eaten regularly, rates of cardiovascular disease are also higher.

---

[4]   *Ibid.*, p. 2

5. The Chinese eat more calories daily than Americans per pound of body weight but suffer little obesity.

6. The average Chinese blood cholesterol level is only 127mg per deciliter compared to 212mg in the United States.

Ninety percent of the Chinese selected for this study were provincials who ate locally raised foods and stuck to a traditional diet. Based on the outcome of this study, the Chinese government is currently taking active steps to keep this traditional diet from giving way to the high-fat diet of the West.

PRESERVING HEALTH & ACHIEVING LONGEVITY WITH A QING DAN DIET

In Chinese there is a saying that before 30 years of age, you cheat disease, but after 30, disease cheats you. In part, this is because, by the mid-30s according to the *Nei Jing*, the spleen and stomach are beginning to decline and grow weak. Most people have the experience that when they were young they could eat and drink anything and seemingly not feel any adverse effects. However, as we get older, we find that we can eat less and less foods without paying the consequences of some adverse reactions. Also, by about 40 years of age, many if not most people put on 10 extra pounds because of the slowing down of the metabolism attendant with aging. In Chinese medicine, fatty tissue is seen as nothing other than excessive phlegm and dampness, and the root of this phlegm and dampness' production is in the Chinese spleen.

Li Chan, author of the famous Ming Dynasty (1368-1644 CE) medical primer, the *Yi Xue Ru Men (Entering the Door of Medicine)*, reiterates the importance of eating a *qing dan* diet if one wishes to keep fit and achieve a healthy old age:

> When a person reaches middle age, their kidney qi is weakening, which, together with intemperance in sexual life, results in vacuity and detriment. Taking supplementing formulas invigorates yang, but also

19

leads to unbearable tidal fevers. Taking (yin) enriching and downbearing medicinals (to reduce evil fire), a person may temporarily feel crisp, but, over time, the middle qi will become even more vacuous and blood will no longer be engendered. Therefore, it is imperative to balance and regulate food and drink, avoiding whatever foods are fried, roasted or toasted, fermented, including alcohol, pickled in soy sauce, or are hot in nature lest they should dry the blood. One should also shun raw, cold fruits and vegetables, lest they damage the spleen. Sweet, bland, thin (or light) foods result in the five flavors automatically supplementing the five viscera. This nourishes the old and enriches the young alike.[5]

---

[5]   Li Chan, *Yi Xue Ru Men* (*Entering the Door of Medicine*), as quoted by Zhang En-qin *et. al.*, *Zhong Yi Yang Sheng Kang Fu Xue* (*The Study of Nourishing Life and Restoring Health in TCM*), Shanghai College of TCM Press, Shanghai, 1990, p. 80

CHAPTER 4

CONGEE

All this being said, you are still probably asking what to eat for breakfast. If my general answer above was a *qing dan* diet, my specific answer here is congee. Congee is a dilute porridge. In China, it is mostly made with rice. However, it can be made with a number of other grains and combinations of grains. In Mandarin Chinese, congee is called *zhou*. In Cantonese, this is pronounced *jook*, and hence the name of this book. Congee is also called *shi fan*, water rice, in Mandarin.

Porridge has also been in the past a traditional breakfast food in the West and especially in the British Isles. Recently, my family and I travelled through England and Scotland, and porridge was served every morning at the bed and breakfasts in which we stayed. However, this porridge was always oatmeal. According to Chinese medicine, oats are very moistening to the lungs. They are a very good food to eat if a person has a dry, chronic sore throat or a chronic, dry cough. However, most Westerners tend to be too damp already, due to eating too many fats, drinking too much fruit juice, and eating too many sweats and dairy products. Therefore, oatmeal porridge is probably not the best morning porridge for Westerners.

In addition, when Westerners eat porridge for breakfast, we usually put either milk or butter on it and some kind of sweetner, such as sugar or honey. These additions make our Western porridges more dampening than is good for most of us.

Chinese congees may be made with a single grain or a combination of grains, beans, vegetables, animal protein, or Chinese medicinal herbs.

Since each type of grain, bean, vegetable, animal protein, or herb has its Chinese medicinal description and use, one can tailor their morning congee to their exact health needs.

OBJECTIONS

1. This doesn't look like Kansas, Toto. That's right. Eating Chinese medicinal congee for breakfast does not look or taste like the typical Western breakfast. But we have already seen that the typical Western breakfast is a dietary disaster, or as some people put it, a heart attack on a plate. There is nothing wrong with eating rice soup and some vegetables in the morning. It is just not what we are used to. However, our insistence that we can only eat a certain type of food for breakfast is the undoing of many an otherwise good diet. In Asia, there is nothing odd or peculiar about eating cooked vegetables for breakfast. It is only our own cultural belief, and probably a fairly recent belief at that, that makes rice soup and vegetables sound unappetizing for breakfast.

During the times that I and my wife have lived and studied in China, we have always preferred the Chinese breakfast (*zhong zao fan*)—with rice congee and vegetables as side dishes—to the so-called Western breakfast (*xi zao fan*) of eggs, toast, and sausage. It is light, yet satisfying. It provides great energy without being heavy and greasy. And when I have studied in China and eaten a diet of nothing but Chinese foods, I have to say I have felt much better than on a typical American diet.

Some time ago I realized that eating a bowl of cereal in the morning swimming in cold, refrigerated milk was making me phlegmy. So I switched to eating congee with some Chinese barley (Job's Tears) to eliminate dampness, some red dates to give the porridge a little flavor and also to supplement my qi and nourish my blood, and some Chinese yam to supplement my spleen and kidneys. On the side, I ate some fresh steamed greens or a selection of different pickled vegetables, some Chinese, some Korean, and some even Kosher. Not only did my phlegm clear up but my digestion improved in general and I lost 6-7 extra pounds I had been carrying around for several years.

In Hong Kong there are congee shops. These are restaurants which are typically open 24 hours a day. Inside there is a huge cauldron of piping hot rice soup. Then there are dishes of chopped vegetables, eggs, and an assortment of meats and seafoods. One takes a bowl and chooses a selection of vegetables, meats, and/or eggs. Then the piping hot rice soup is ladled into the bowl, immediately poaching the meat, fish, or eggs and the vegetables. Thus, the ingredients are cooked by the soup just enough to make them more easily digestible but not enough to lose valuable enzymes and vitamins—and all without the use of cooking oils or fats. This is a cuisine all of its own, and a very nutritious, delicious, and healthy one at that.

2. I don't have time to cook porridge in the morning. I have to get to work. Me too! That's the beauty of congee for us busy Westerners. Simply go out and buy a crock pot or slow cooker. These are electrical, free-standing, so-called Dutch ovens. Most people use them to cook pot roasts, stews, soups, and chilies. You put the rice and water plus whatever other grains, beans, or Chinese herbs you want in the pot, turn it on low, and leave it to simmer over night. In the morning when you wake, your breakfast is ready to eat. Just spoon it out, season to taste, and dig in.

THE MEDICINAL BENEFITS OF CONGEE

Most of the time, Chinese congee is made with rice. Therefore, *shi fan* or water rice has all the benefits of eating rice itself. It supplements the middle burner and boosts the qi, fortifies the spleen and harmonizes the stomach. However, because congee is eaten as a 100° soup in a form immediately suitable for digestion and absorption, rice congee particularly benefits the stomach and intestines. Because it is cooked with so much water, congee helps moisten the fluids of the stomach and intestines which tend to become depleted in old age and due to chronic disease. However, it does this without engendering dampness and phlegm. Ge Hong, a famous Daoist saint and doctor of the Eastern Jin Dynasty (265-420 CE) stated that, "To prolong life, it is essential to keep the stomach and intestines clear,"[6] and congee does just that. Because it is light and easy to digest, it does not overburden the stomach and intestines with heavy, hard-to-digest foods.

In fact, eating congee is so beneficial to the health that many ancient and contemporary Chinese books on health preservation and boosting longevity stress "eating congee (shi zhou)" as a special practice. Li Jing of the Qing Dynasty (1644-1911 CE) believed that congee "is able to smooth the stomach qi and engender fluids and humors."[7] In the *Lei Xiu Yao Jue (Rhymed Essentials for Cultivation [of Longevity])*, it says, "Drinking 1 *hu* of wine is not as (good as) eating till full one congee."[8] And Lu You of the Southern Song Dynasty (960-1280 CE) said:

> Everyone wishes to live long, but they do not know that the means to prolonging life are in front of their eyes. I obtained from Wan Qiu a simple method. It suggests that eating congee can make one a divine immortal.[9]

Cao Ting-dong, also of the Qing Dynasty, compiled a congee cookbook for the elderly to help them keep fit. In it he says, "Old people who eat gruel all day, not sticking to fixed times, are also able to keep their body strong and fortified and enjoy great longevity."[10] Likewise, Xu

---

[6] Ge Hong, *Bao Pu Zi Nei Pian (Bao Pu Zi's Inner Writings)*, as quoted by Zhang En-qin *et. al.*, *Zhong Yi Yang Sheng Kang Fu Xue (The Study of Nourishing Life and Restoring Health in TCM)*, Shanghai College of TCM Press, Shanghai, 1990, p.

[7] *Ibid.*, p. 104

[8] *Ibid.*, p. 104

[9] *Ibid.*, p. 104

[10] *Ibid.*, p. 104

Zong-heng of the Qing Dynasty advised people to eat congee before dawn:

> Cook the congee until the water and rice become indivisible and eat before the fifth watch (*i.e.*, dawn). It is sweet and beautiful to the mouth and entering the abdomen it feels cool and refreshing... For the most delicious food under heaven, there is nothing which exceeds grains and also nothing which goes beyond bland food.[11]

In particular, rice congee is beneficial for anyone with a weak digestion. This includes babies and infants, anyone who is ill, anyone recuperating from a prolonged or serious disease, anyone who is constitutionally weak or weakened from overtaxation, and the elderly. In an ancient Chinese classic, it is said:

> When treating a poor vacuity patient, use a thick rice soup. This is as good as a decoction of Ginseng.[12]

It also says, "Ordinary rice porridge is a miraculous substance for the growth and development of the body, and sweet rice is a unique agent for warming and nurturing the spleen and stomach."[13] Thus congee can and should be the first food given to infants after breast milk. And it is just as appropriate for those in their last years of life. Congee is so healthful and nutritious that the Buddha had this to say about it:

> It confers 10 things on those who eat it: life and beauty, ease and strength. It dispels hunger, thirst, and wind. It cleanses the bladder. It digests food. This food is praised by the Well-farer.[14]

---

[11] *Ibid.*, p. 104

[12] Quoted by Wang Lu-chu, "Medicinal Porridge", *Journal of the American College of TCM*, San Francisco, 1985, #4, p. 51

[13] *Ibid.*, p. 51

[14] Shakyamuni Buddha, Makavagga, *Vinanaya Pitaka (Book of the Discipline)*, trans. by I. B. Harner, London, 1951, Vol. IV, p. 302

In Chinese medicine, the prognosis of any disease is based on three things: spirit, stomach qi, and root. Spirit refers to the heart spirit which is nourished by qi. Root refers to the kidney essence which is also nourished by qi. Thus Li Dong-yuan said:

> Qi is the forefather of spirit and essence is the child of qi. (Thus) qi is the root of essence and spirit. Great is qi! When qi accumulates, it produces essence. When essence accumulates, it renders spirit wholesome.[15]

The qi that Li is referring to is the stomach or middle qi, the postnatal root of qi and blood production. Once stomach qi fails, we can no longer make new qi and blood postnatally and thus must decline and die. That is why Cai Jing-feng, author of *Eating Your Way to Health: Dietotherapy in Traditional Chinese Medicine*, can say:

> It is believed in traditional Chinese medicine that when the vital energy of the stomach is depleted, the disease will be incurable, and that is why rice porridge is considered to be the most fundamental of dietotherapeutic foods.[16]

A SHORT HISTORY OF CONGEE IN CHINESE MEDICINE

The first written records of Chinese medicinal porridges come from the Ma Wang Dui tombs dating from the Han Dynasty (206 BCE-220 CE). In these tombs were found 14 volumes of medical books. Included in these books are prescriptions for medicinal porridge for the treatment of snake bite and anal itching. In all probability, these prescriptions date back to the Spring and Autumn and Warring States periods (770-221 BCE).

---

[15] Li Dong-yuan, *Pi Wei Lun (Treatise on the Spleen and Stomach)*, trans. by Yang Shou-zhong and Li Jian-yong, Blue Poppy Press, Boulder, CO, 1993, p. 261

[16] Cai Jing-feng, *Eating Your Way to Health: Dietotherapy in Traditional Chinese Medicine,* Foreign Languages Press, Beijing, 1988, p. 28

Nevertheless, it was not until the Tang and Song Dynasties that Chinese medicinal porridges were used extensively by professional practitioners for the treatment of disease. It is likely, however, that medicinal porridges have a much longer folk or unrecorded history. It was only in the Tang and Song Dynasties that Confucian scholar-doctors began writing about the use of congee in their practice. Since that time, the number of Chinese writings on this subject has continually increased. In the Tang Dynasty (618-907 CE), the great Chinese doctor Sun Si-miao included several congee recipes in his *Qian Jin Yao Fang (Prescriptions [Worth a] Thousand [Pieces of] Gold)*, including Milk Congee (*Niu Nai Zhou*), Phragmites Congee (*Lu Gen Zhou*), and Trichosanthes Congee (*Tian Hua Fen Zhou*). In the *Tai Ping Sheng Hui Fang (Supreme Peace, Holy, Benevolent Prescriptions)* compiled in 992 CE by Wang Huai-yin, there are 129 medicinal porridge formulas, many of them still in use today and many of them found in this book.

In the Ming Dynasty (1368-1644 CE), Li Shi-zhen, in his monumental *Ben Cao Gang Mu (Great Outline of the Materia Medica)*, gives formulas for 62 medicinal porridges with their functions and indications. In the Qing Dynasty, both medical practitioners and scholars studying, using, and writing on medicinal porridges increased in large number. For instance, Zhang Xi-shung created Dioscorea Congee (*Shan Yao Zhou*), Pearl & Jade Two Treasures Congee (*Zhen Yu Er Bao Zhou*), Three Treasures Congee (*San Bao Zhou*), Dioscorea & Pinellia Congee (*Shan Yao Ban Xia Zhou*), and Dioscorea & Egg Yolk Congee (*Shan Yao Ji Zi Huang Zhou*). Today, according to Wang Shui, Lu Zhong-ling, and Chu Nong in their article "Medicinal Porridge" published in *The Journal of the American College of Traditional Chinese Medicine*, "Many noted contemporary Chinese doctors always make a point of using medicinal porridge for the prevention and treatment of various diseases..."[17]

---

[17] Wang, Lu, Chu, *op. cit.*, p. 49

CONTRAINDICATIONS TO CONGEE

Since congee can be made with any number of grains or beans as its base, there are no contraindications to congee as such. However, there are contraindications to some of the grains and beans that are used to make congee and the first is rice. Rice is also a diuretic. In TCM terms, it disinhibits water and thus promotes urination. Therefore, people who suffer from polyuria due to yang and qi vacuity should not eat a lot of rice congee. Likewise, aduki beans and mung beans are also diuretics. These can also worsen vacuity in patients with polyuria due to vacuity. As Li Dong-yuan says:

> Rice congee, (steamed) rice, mung beans, red beans, and fermented beans with salt are all bland percolators and urine disinhibitors. (In case of) frequent urination, disinhibition of urination is not allowed. What's more, (such disinhibition) greatly drains the yang qi...[18]

GENERAL DIRECTIONS ON MAKING CONGEE

Although the various recipes given in this book for different types of Chinese medicinal porridges give their own directions, a general direction for making congee is to use 1 part rice to 5, 6, or even 7 or 8 parts water. Usually, one makes rice by cooking 1 part rice to 2 parts water. However, with congee, we want to end up with a thin gruel, soup, or porridge. If one is eating the porridge alone, they may want it to be a little thicker. However, if you intend to poach an egg or some seafood in the piping hot liquid congee, it needs to be thinner and thus made with more water. First bring the water to a boil and then turn the heat down to a slow simmer. If one uses a crock pot or slow cooker, the porridge can be left to cook overnight. One can also cook the congee on a stove and, in that case, can cook it in 2-4 hours.

---

[18] Li Dong-yuan, *op. cit.*, p. 257

SPECIFIC INSTRUCTIONS
FOR MAKING MEDICINAL CONGEES

Medicinal congees are made by adding Chinese medicinals to various grains and beans and cooking these into porridge. Some of these Chinese medicinals, such as Fructus Zizyphi Jujubae (*i.e.* Chinese Red Dates, *Hong Zao* or *Da Zao*) and Semen Pini (*i.e.*, Pine Nuts, *Song Zi Ren*), are fruits and seeds and are tasty additions which can be cooked whole in the porridge and eaten along with the porridge in the same way that Westerners might add almonds or raisins to oatmeal.

Other Chinese medicinals are not so tasty or not that nice to eat whole. Therefore, there are several ways of making Chinese medicinal porridges that are nevertheless palatable. Sometimes, dried roots or other starchy medicinals, such as Radix Puerariae Lobatae (*i.e.*, Kudzu Root, *Ge Gen*), Radix Dioscoreae Oppositae (*i.e.*, Chinese Yam, *Shan Yao*), or Sclerotium Poriae Cocos (*Fu Ling*), are ground into powder and added to the cooking porridge as if they were a grain or flour. The resulting porridges are smooth, creamy, and quite delicious.

Other times, Chinese medicinals, such as Semen Citri (*i.e.*, Orange Seeds, *Ju He*), are cooked in the congee but are removed prior to eating. Another common way of making medicinal congees is to first decoct the Chinese medicinals—commonly roots, barks, flowers, or leaves—remove the dregs, and reserve the liquid. This liquid is then added to the grain, usually rice, along with additional water and then cooked into porridge. That way, one does not have to eat bitter-tasting pieces of roots and bark.

THE TYPES OF GRAINS MOST COMMONLY
USED IN CHINESE MEDICINAL CONGEES

The majority of medicinal congees included in this book are made from rice. However, a number of other grains are also used. When specifying rice, there are two major kinds mentioned. These are *jing mi* and *da mi*. *Jing mi* refers to polished round grain rice, while *da mi* refers to polished long grain rice. However, I have simply referred to these as polished rice, meaning white rice. In one instance, brown or unpolished rice is specified. This is called *cao mi* or literally coarse, rough, *i.e.*, unpolished, rice.

Other grains used in the formulas described in this book include millet, *xiao mi*, *shu mi*, and *su mi*; wheat, *xiao mai*; sorghum, *gao liang mi*; Job's tears barley, *yi yi ren*; regular barley, *da mai*; and corn or *yu mi*. The main beans used in making the formulas herein include aduki beans, *chi xiao dou*; mung beans, *lu dou*; and black soybeans, *hei dou*. All these ingredients, except for the Job's tears barley, can usually be purchased at well-stocked health food stores.

CONGEE & TRADITIONAL CHINESE MEDICINALS IN PRACTICE

In Chinese medicine there is no hard and fast line between food and medicine. There is even the saying in Chinese, "*Yao shi tong yuan,* medicine and food have a common source." Most traditional Chinese medicinals are herbs, roots, barks, fruits, seeds, and nuts. Some Chinese medicinals are made from animal products, while others are made from minerals. Many of the herbs, fruits, seeds, nuts, and animal products are also foods eaten as a part of the Chinese diet. Even the standard method of medicinal administration in TCM, the *tang* or decoction, means literally nothing more than soup. Therefore, Chinese medicinal porridges can be seen either as especially healthy foods or as medicinal prescriptions, and they should be prescribed on the basis of a TCM pattern discrimination just as if writing a prescription for a medicinal decoction.

So then the question is, should one use both decoctions and medicinal porridges or only one or the other? The answer entirely depends on the situation at hand. If used for disease prevention and health preservation, one may choose to only use medicinal porridges on a daily basis and not drink Chinese medicinal decoctions. However, if one become more seriously ill, then drinking a strong Chinese medicinal decoction until one's health returns to normal probably makes more sense. That does not mean that the person cannot also eat a medicinal porridge at the same time. They can and usually should. Almost anyone who is sick can benefit from a simple rice congee. And if some medicinals appropriate to one's TCM pattern discrimination are also added, so much the better.

In addition, there are cases where prescribing Chinese medicinals as a medicinal congee is the best course of treatment. For instance, in the case of high fever in a patient with a weak spleen and stomach, one may wish to prescribe Gypsum Fibrosum (*Shi Gao*) to clear heat and recede the fever. However, because Gypsum is very cold and enters the stomach channel, the use of Gypsum in such a case may be contraindicated. In that case, one can make a medicinal porridge with Gypsum and rice. The Gypsum will clear the heat and the rice will protect and nourish the stomach qi and fluids.

In a similar way, there are certain TCM decoctions which classically are supposed to be taken with rice congee. For instance, Zhang Zhong-jing, writing in the *Shang Han Lun (Treatise on Damage by Cold)* about *Gui Zhi Tang* (Ramulus Cinnamomi Decoction) says, "Wait for a short time (after having taken the herbal decoction) and then take 1 or more *sheng* of hot congee to institute a joint action."[19] As Zhou Feng-wu explains:

> The administration of hot dilute porridge aids the stomach qi, provides substance for the *ying* and *wei*, engenders fluids, and assists in the distribution of fluids in the middle burner. It also carries the hidden evil with the sweet towards the exterior. It is to be noted that the drinking of hot dilute porridge is one of the essential components of *Gui Zhi Tang*.[20]

---

[19] Zhou Feng-wu, "The Indications of Decoction Ramulus Cinnamomi Composite," trans. by C. S. Cheung and M. Hirano, *Journal of American College of TCM*, San Francisco, 1983, #1, p. 11

[20] *Ibid.*, p. 11

There are also some other situations when prescribing a Chinese medicinal porridge makes sense in Western practice. First, for those just learning Chinese herbal medicine, using simple, one and two ingredient medicinal congees is a way to ease into the practice of Chinese herbal medicine. There is a lot of information to keep in mind when writing a prescription with 15-18 ingredients in it. One needs to know the individual characteristics of each ingredient and then how they will work synergistically in a formula. When using only 1-2 ingredients, there is a lot less to keep in mind.

Secondly, acupuncturists who do not regularly prescribe Chinese herbal medicine may find it useful in some cases to prescribe 1-2 ingredient medicinal porridges to help extend and reinforce the benefits of acupuncture. Many of the ingredients are foods which are available at health food stores and Oriental specialty food shops. Therefore, the acupuncturist would not have to put in a large dispensary but merely write down the instructions and where to purchase the ingredients.

Third, and in the same way, patients with chronic conditions who are being treated with fairly low potency pills and soluble powdered extracts may benefit by eating simple Chinese medicinal porridges. In this way they can get more effect than by just taking the pills alone, but porridges are easier and more palatable to take than straight Chinese herbal decoctions.

PURCHASING CHINESE MEDICINALS

Readers in the United States can order most of the Chinese medicinals mentioned in this book from:

Spring Wind Herb Company
2315 Fourth St
Berkeley, CA 94710
Tel. 510-849-1820
Fax: 510-849-4886
Orders: 800-588-4883

This company sells Chinese herbs by mail order and customers can order using either the Pinyin romanization of the Chinese name or the Latin pharmacological name. (I give both in this book.) This company goes to great lengths to import and sell Chinese herbs free from pesticides, fumigants, bleaches, and other chemical contaminants.

Other companies in the United States that sell Chinese herbs by mail are:

China Herb Co.
6333 Wayne Ave.
Philadelphia, PA 19144
Tel. 215-843-5864, 1-800-221-4372; Fax 215-849-3338

Mayway Corp.
1338 Cypress St.
Oakland, CA 94607
Tel. 510-208-3113

North South China Herbs Co.
1556 Stockton Street
San Francisco, CA 94133
Tel. 415-421-4907

Nuherbs Co.
3820 Penniman Avenue
Oakland, CA 94619
Tel. 415-534-4372; 1-800-233-4307

For those in the United Kingdom, most of the medicinals in this book can be ordered from:

Acumedic Ltd.
101-105 Camden High Street
London NW1 7JN
Tel. 071-388-6704/5783; Fax 071-387-5766

East West Herb Shop
3 Neals Yard
Covent Garden, London WC2H 9DP
Tel. 071-379-1312; Fax 071-379-4414

Harmony Acupuncture Supplies Center
629 High Road Leytonstone
London E11 4PA
Tel. 081-518-7337; Fax 081-518-7338

Mayway Herbal Emporium
40 Sapcote Trading Estate, Dudden Hill Lane
London NW10 2DJ
Tel. 081-459-1812; Fax 081-459-1727

For those in Europe, most of the medicinals in this book can be ordered from:

Homeofar n.v.
Hugo Verriestlaan 63
8500 Kortrijk, Belgium

Tai Yang Chinese Herb Store
Elverdingsestr. 90A
8900 Ieper, Belgium
Tel. 057-21-86-69; Fax 057-21-97-78

Apotheek Gouka
Goenelaan 111
3114 CE Schiedam, Netherlands
Tel. 010-426-46-33; Fax 010-473-08-45

And for those in Australia, most of the medicinals in this book can be ordered from:

Chinaherb
29A Albion St.
Surry Hills, NSW 2010
Tel. 02-281-2122

WHERE TO FIND OUT MORE INFORMATION ON INDIVIDUAL CHINESE MEDICINALS

When prescribing Chinese medicinal congees, as when prescribing any Chinese herbal formula, one should know what the purpose and functions of each ingredient in the formula are before prescribing that formula. Only in possession of this knowledge can one be sure a given formula fits a specific patient. If one wants to find out more information on any of the individual medicinals comprising the formulas in this book, most of these are discussed in Bensky and Gamble's *Chinese Herbal Medicine: Materia Medica* published by Eastland Press, Seattle, WA. Those that are not included in that standard text will typically be found in Hong-yen Hsu's *Oriental Materia Medica: A Concise Guide* published by the Oriental Healing Arts Institute, Long Beach, CA.

For the Chinese medicinal descriptions of most of the individual foods described in this book, the reader is referred to Honora Lee Wolfe's and my *Prince Wen Hui's Cook, Chinese Dietary Therapy* published by Paradigm Publications, Brookline, MA.

CHAPTER 5

USING THIS BOOK

PATTERN DISCRIMINATION

TCM as a distinct style of Chinese medicine bases its treatments on pattern discrimination more than on disease diagnosis. This means that two patients with the same disease but different patterns will receive different formulas, while two patients with different diseases but the same pattern will receive the same formula. This holds true with the prescription and administration of Chinese medicinal congees. This means that, although the congees in this book are arranged under disease categories, such as high blood pressure and diabetes mellitus, a congee listed under a different disease may also be used to treat the disease in question. Thus the reader will see when looking at the indications of a congee under high blood pressure that it also may treat high cholesterol and even premature greying of the hair as long as these different diseases are associated with a single pattern. This is because these congees, like other TCM medicinal formulas, are not disease specific but pattern specific.

Professional TCM practitioners should have no problem identifying the patterns appropriate to each congee in this book. This can be done by looking at the functions of each individual ingredient as discussed above and also by looking at the functions listed for each congee as a whole. If a congee clears heat and disinhibits dampness and is indicated for cystitis, then it is specifically damp heat in the lower burner cystitis that this congee treats. Therefore, the congee under question does not treat all types of cystitis or bladder infections, but only one type, the damp heat type. If, in fact, the patient is suffering from a qi vacuity pattern cystitis, the damp heat clearing and eliminating congee might very well make that patient worse. This is because heat-clearing and dampness-disinhibiting are species of draining and a qi vacuity requires supplementation. Thus the erroneous choice of this formula in the case of qi vacuity cystitis would result in further evacuating what is already vacuous.

The prescription of medicinals based on TCM patterns, such as stomach cold, lung heat, yin vacuity, and kidney qi not securing, is not only the foundation of TCM as a system but the very thing that makes TCM both safe and effective. Prescribing on the basis of a pattern discrimination is nothing other than assuring that a given formula fits the totality of the patient. Because it fits the entire patient in all their manifestations, it not only treats the disease or major complaint but harmonizes and balances the patient's entire condition. Therefore, with correctly prescribed TCM formulas there is healing without side effects.

FINDING A TCM PRACTITIONER

However, this methodology which makes TCM as a style of medicine so safe and effective must be learned professionally. Since it has little to do with the disease categories of modern Western medicine or with the theories of modern Western biology, the Western lay reader interested in availing themselves of the treatments contained in this book is strongly advised to seek out a professional practitioner of TCM. Since most TCM practitioners in the West practice under the heading of acupuncture, that is where the prospective patient should first look. In the United States of America, prospective patients can look in the Yellow Pages under acupuncture, or they may call their state Department of Health or Department of Regulatory Agencies to find out if acupuncture and Chinese medicine are legal in that state and, if so, for a list of licensed or registered acupuncturists. Once armed with the phone numbers of some local acupuncturists, the prospective patient should then ask if a) the practitioner is trained specifically in TCM and b) do they practice Chinese herbal medicine and dietary therapy.

If a person is already a patient of an acupuncturist or TCM practitioner, they may ask their practitioner to mark the congees in this book that would be most helpful for re-establishing balance and restoring health to their condition. Lay people interested in reading further about Traditional Chinese Medicine are referred to Ted Kaptchuk's *The Web That Has No Weaver* published by Congdon & Weed of New York.

USING THE GENERAL INDEX

Professional practitioners using this book should look not only under the disease categories which form the subsections of the treatment formulary chapters of this book but should also look up the disease or symptom under question in the general index at the rear of this book. This way, they will find a greater selection of formulas for each disease. In a few instances, I have included a single congee under more than one disease category. However, to save paper and trees, we have made the general index as user-friendly and complete as possible.

Bon appetit!

BOOK II

TREATMENT FORMULARY

17) High Blood Pressure
18) High Cholesterol
19) Coronary Heart Dz
20) Congestive Heart Failure
21) Chronic Low Blood Pressure
22) Wind Stroke
23) Neurosthenia
24) Hepatitis / Lv. + Sp. Hypertrophy
25) Cirrhosis
26) Superficial Edema, Ascites
27) Diarrhea
28) Dysentery
29) Constipation
30) Incontinenca / Kid ae xu
31) Nephritis / Renal Tubercalosis
32) Strangury Dz / dribbling / cystitis
33) Impotensy

34) Spermotorrhea
35) Low Back / knee pain
36) Testicalar pain / swelling
37) Night Sweats

IMPORTANT MESSAGE

FOR _____

DATE _____ TIME _____ A.M. P.M.

M _____

OF _____

PHONE _____
AREA CODE / NUMBER / EXTENSION

☐ FAX

☐ MOBILE _____
AREA CODE / NUMBER / TIME TO CALL

TELEPHONED		PLEASE CALL	
CAME TO SEE YOU		WILL CALL AGAIN	
WANTS TO SEE YOU		RUSH	
RETURNED YOUR CALL		SPECIAL ATTENTION	

MESSAGE _____

_____

_____

_____

_____

SIGNED _____

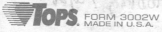

TOPS FORM 3002W
MADE IN U.S.A.

Int. Medicin

Colds + Flu

Summer heat

1) Fever

2) Cough

5) Pneumonia

6) Coughing + Panting
    Asthma

7) Pulmonary Tuberculosis

8) Meningitis

9) Indigestion

10) Vomiting / Hiccups

11) Stomach pain

12) Stomach + Duodenal Ulcers

13) upper digest tract Bleeding

14) Thyroid Hypertrophy / Lymphadenopathy

15) Diabetis Mellitus

16) Anemia

IMPORTANT MESSAGE

FOR _____

DATE _____ TIME _____ A.M. / P.M.

M _____

OF _____

PHONE _____
AREA CODE   NUMBER   EXTENSION

☐ FAX

☐ MOBILE _____
AREA CODE   NUMBER   TIME TO CALL

TELEPHONED		PLEASE CALL	
CAME TO SEE YOU		WILL CALL AGAIN	
WANTS TO SEE YOU		RUSH	
RETURNED YOUR CALL		SPECIAL ATTENTION	

MESSAGE _____

_____

_____

_____

_____

SIGNED _____

CHAPTER 1

INTERNAL MEDICINE
(NEI KE)

1
Colds & Flu (*Gan Mao*)

Scallion & Glutinous Rice Congee
(*Cong Bai Nuo Mi Zhou*)

Functions: Effuses the exterior, resolves toxins

Indications: The initial stages of an external attack resulting in generalized aching and pain, aversion to cold, fear of chill, and other such symptoms

Ingredients: Herba Allii Fistulosi (*i.e.*, Scallion, *Cong Bai*), 5 whole ones, raw Rhizoma Zingiberis (*i.e.*, Fresh Ginger, *Sheng Jiang*), 15g, Semen Oryzae Glutinosae (*i.e.*, Glutinous Rice, *Nuo Mi*), 100g

Method of preparation & administration: First cook the rice into a porridge. Then mash the scallions and ginger into a pulp. Add to the congee and simmer, then take. Discharging sweat results in a cure.

Glutinous Rice & Scallion Congee
(*Nuo Mi Cong Zhou*)

Functions: Courses wind and scatters cold

Indications: Wind cold external invasion and stuffy nose

Ingredients: Semen Oryzae Glutinosae (*i.e.*, Glutinous Rice, *Nuo Mi*), 100g, Herba Allii Fistulosi (*i.e.*, Scallion, *Cong Bai*), several roots

Method of preparation & administration: First cook the glutinous rice into a porridge. While still hot, add the scallions and briefly bring to a boil. Eat on an empty stomach. Discharging a slight sweat brings improvement.

Xanthium Seed Congee
(Cang Er Zi Zhou)

Functions: Dispels wind and scatters cold, brightens the eyes and ears, opens the portal of the nose

Indications: Wind cold headache, stuffy nose, tooth aching and pain, wind, cold, damp *bi* pain, etc,

Ingredients: Fructus Xanthii (*Cang Er Zi*) 15g, Semen Oryzae Sativae (*i.e.*, Polished Rice, *Jing Mi*), 50g

Method of preparation & administration: First stir-fry the Xanthium seeds till yellow. Then decoct in 200ml of water down to 100ml, remove the dregs, and reserve the liquid. Add this to the rice plus 400ml of water and cook into porridge. Eat warm 2 times per day.

Schizonepeta Congee
(Jing Jie Zhou)

Functions: Relieves the exterior, courses wind, and scatters cold

Indications: Wind cold common cold and flu

Ingredients: Spica Seu Flos Schizonepetae Tenuifoliae (*Jing Jie Sui*), 9g, Herba Menthae (*Bo He*), 3g, Semen Praeparatum Sojae (*Dan Dou Chi*), 9g, Semen Oryzae Sativae (*i.e.*, Polished Rice, *Jing Mi*), 100g

Method of preparation & administration: Decoct the first 3 ingredients in water for only 5-7 minutes, remove the dregs, and reserve the liquid. Then make porridge from the rice and add this liquid. Take warm 2 times per day.

Mint & Chrysanthemum
(Bo Ju Zhou)

Functions: Relieves the exterior, dispels wind, and clears heat

Indications: Wind heat common cold and flu

Ingredients: Herba Menthae (*Bo He*), 9g, Flos Chrysanthemi Morifolii (*Ju Hua*), 9g, Folium Mori Albi (*Sang Ye*), 6g, Herba Lophatheri Gracilis (*Dan Zhu Ye*), 6g, Semen Oryzae Sativae (*i.e.*, Polished Rice, *Jing Mi*), 100g

Method of preparation & administration: Decoct the first 4 ingredients in water for 5-7 minutes, remove the dregs, and reserve the liquid. Then cook the rice into porridge and add this liquid. Take 2 times per day.

Burdock Seed Congee
(Niu Bang Zi Zhou)

Functions: Courses and scatters wind heat, resolves toxins and recedes rashes, disinhibits the throat and disperses swelling, brightens the eyes

Indications: External invasion of wind heat, cough with common cold, phlegmy cough which is not crisp (sounding), swollen, sore throat, measles rash which will not recede smoothly, water swelling, constipation, etc.

Ingredients: Fructus Arctii Lappae (*i.e.*, Burdock Seeds, *Niu Bang Zi*), 15g, Semen Oryzae Sativae (*i.e.*, Polished Rice, *Jing Mi*), 50g, Granulated Sugar (*Bing Tang*), a suitable amount

Method of preparation & administration: First decoct the burdock seeds in 200ml of water down to 100ml, remove the dregs, and reserve the liquid. Add this and 400ml more water to the rice and sugar and cook into porridge. Eat warm 2 times per day.

Contraindications: Stomach cold, qi vacuity

Double Flower Congee
(*Shuang Hua Zhou*)

Functions: Clears heat and resolves toxins, attacks germs and disperses inflammation

Indications: Wind heat common cold and flu, pneumonia, upper respiratory tract infection, acute bacterial dysentery, hot toxin ulcers, sore, swollen throat, acute inflammation of the eyes, suppurative inflammations of the skin and exterior

Ingredients: Flos Lonicerae Japonicae (*Yin Hua*), 30g, Semen Oryzae Sativae (*i.e.*, Polished Rice, *Jing Mi*), 30g

Method of preparation & administration: First decoct the Lonicera flowers, remove the dregs, and reserve 150ml of the liquid. Next cook the rice into porridge in 300ml of water and add this 150ml of liquid. Take warm 2 times per day in the morning and evening.

2
Summerheat Disease (*Shu Bing*)

Dolichos & Lotus Leaf Congee
(*Bian He Zhou*)

Functions: Disperses summerheat and resolves fever, harmonizes the stomach and thickens the intestines, stops diarrhea

Indications: Summerheat fever. Eating regularly during the summer boosts and fortifies the constitution.

Ingredients: Semen Dolichos Lablabis (*Bai Bian Dou*), 50g, Granulated Sugar (*Bing Tang*), 30g, fresh Folium Nelumbinis Nuciferae (*Xian He Ye*), 1 small piece, Semen Oryzae Sativae (*i.e.*, Polished Rice, *Da Mi*), 50g

Method of preparation & administration: With clean water, first wash and soak the white rice. Then add the Dolichos and extra water and cook over a small fire until this becomes a pasty consistency. Then add the granulated sugar and lotus leaves and cook for another 20 minutes. Because of the sweet flavor of the lotus leaves, this is an ideal food.

Mung Bean Congee
(*Lu Dou Zhou*)

Functions: Clears summerheat and engenders fluids, resolves toxins and disperses swelling

Indications: Summerheat fever and vexatious thirst, toxic ulcers and swellings. Eating in the summer helps prevent summerheat stroke.

Ingredients: Semen Phaseoli Mungonis (*i.e.*, Mung Beans, *Lu Dou*), 50g, Semen Oryzae Sativae (*i.e.*, Polished Rice, *Jing Mi*), 250g, Granulated Sugar (*Bing Tang*), a suitable amount

Method of preparation & administration: Make into porridge as usual and add sugar to taste.

Coix & Dolichos Congee
(*Yi Mi Bian Dou Zhou*)

Functions: Clears summerheat and eliminates dampness

Indications: Summerheat stroke with dampness

Ingredients: Semen Coicis Lachryma-jobi (*Yi Mi*), 30g, Semen Dolichos Lablabis (*Bai Bian Dou*), 30g, Semen Oryzae Sativae (*i.e.*, Polished Rice, *Jing Mi*), 100g

Method of preparation & administration: Make into porridge as usual and eat 2 times per day.

Agastaches Congee
(*Huo Xiang Zhou*)

Functions: Scatters summerheat qi, wards off malignant qi

Indications: External invasion of summerheat dampness evils, fever, chest oppression, devitalized appetite, heavy head, bodily fatigue, nausea, vomiting, diarrhea, abdominal distention and pain, a thick, slimy tongue coating, bad breath, etc.

Ingredients: Dry, powdered Herba Agastachis Seu Pogostemi (*Huo Xiang*), 10g, Semen Oryzae Sativae (*i.e.*, Polished Rice, *Jing Mi*), 50g

Method of preparation & administration: Add 500ml to the rice and cook into porridge. Mix in the Agastaches powder and cook a short time more. Allow to sit for 5 minutes after taking off the fire. Eat warm 2 times per day.

Chinese Quince Congee
(*Mu Gua Zhou*)

Functions: Soothes the sinews and quickens the network vessels, harmonizes the stomach and transforms dampness

Indications: Summerheat and dampness vomiting and diarrhea, twisted sinews of the lower leg, contracture and spasm of the sinews and vessels, foot qi and superficial edema, wind, cold, damp *bi*, etc.

Ingredients: Fresh Fructus Chaenomelis Lagenariae (*Xian Mu Gua*), 1 whole one (or 20g of dry Chaenomeles), Semen Oryzae Sativae (*i.e.*, Polished Rice, *Jing Mi*), 50g, White Sugar (*Bai Tang*), a small amount

Method of preparation & administration: First cut the quince into pieces. Add 200ml of water and decoct down to 100ml. Remove the dregs and reserve the liquid. Add the rice, sugar, and another 400ml of water and cook into porridge. Take 2-3 times per day warm.

Stinking Herb Congee
(*Chou Cao Zhou*)

Functions: Cools the blood and resolves toxins, disperses and eliminates summerheat qi

Indications: Damage by summerheat, hot skin lesions, dizziness, distended brain

Ingredients: Herba Rutae Graveolentis (*Chou Cao*), 50g, Semen Oryzae Sativae (*i.e.*, Polished Rice, *Jing Mi*)

Method of preparation & administration: Cook into porridge as usual and eat.

Dispel Dampness Congee
(*Qu Shi Zhou*)

Functions: Dispels dampness, disinhibits water, secures the intestines

Indications: Summerheat and heat leading to inhibited urination, stomach stagnation and discomfort

Ingredients: Semen Phaseoli Calcarati (*i.e.*, Aduki Beans, *Chi Xiao Dou*), Semen Dolichos Lablabis (*Bai Bian Dou*), Semen Coicis Lachryma-jobi (*Yi Mi*), Semen Euryalis Ferocis (*Qian Shi*), Sichuan Rhizoma Dioscoreae Hypoglaucae (*Chuan Bi Xie*), Sclerotium Rubrum

Poriae Cocos (*Chi Fu Ling*), Flos Gossampini Malabaricae (*Mu Mian Hua*), Medulla Junci Effusi (*Deng Xin Cao*), 10-15g each

Method of preparation & administration: Add water and cook into porridge as usual.

3
Fever (*Fa Re*)

Gypsum Congee
(*Shi Gao Zhou*)

Functions: Clears heat and discharges fire, eliminates vexation and stops thirst

Indications: High fever in the elderly, clouding of consciousness, delirious speech, vexation and agitation, restlessness, oral thirst, excessive drinking, lung heat panting, stomach fire toothache in the elderly, headache, sore throat, etc.

Ingredients: Raw Gypsum Fibrosum (*Sheng Shi Gao*), 200g, Semen Oryzae Sativae (*i.e.*, Polished Rice, *Jing Mi*), 100g

Method of preparation & administration: First grind the Gypsum into powder. Then decoct in 300ml of water down to 200ml. Remove the dregs and reserve the liquid. Add this to the rice plus 600ml of water and cook into porridge. Eat this each day in the morning and afternoon.

4
Cough (*Ke Sou*)

Mustard Congee
(*Jie Cai Zhou*)

Functions: Diffuses the lungs and sweeps away phlegm, warms the center and boosts the stomach, resolves the exterior and disinhibits urination

Indications: Cold rheum internally exuberant, cough, phlegm panting (*i.e.*, asthma), or coughing and vomiting phlegm, chest and diaphragm fullness and oppression, inhibited urination, chronic bronchitis

Ingredients: Fresh Herba Sinapis Junceae (*i.e.*, Mustard Greens, *Xian Jie Cai*), 60g, Semen Oryzae Sativae (*i.e.*, Polished Rice, *Jing Mi*), 100g

Method of preparation & administration: First wash and cut the mustard greens. Then cook these and the rice in water to make porridge as usual. Eat warm 2 times per day.

Perilla Leaf & Apricot Seed Congee
(*Su Ye Xing Ren Zhou*)

Functions: Relieves the exterior and transforms phlegm, downbears qi and stops cough

Indications: Wind cold cough and bronchitis

Ingredients: Folium Perillae Frutescentis (*Su Ye*), 9g, Semen Pruni Armeniacae (*Xing Ren*), 9g, Pericarpium Citri Reticulatae (*Chen Pi*), 6g, Semen Oryzae Sativae (*i.e.*, Polished Rice, *Jing Mi*), 50g

Method of preparation & administration: Decoct the first 3 ingredients in water, remove the dregs, and reserve the liquid. Then make porridge with the rice using this liquid and eat.

Orange Peel Congee
(Ju Hong Zhou)

Functions: Eliminates dampness and transforms phlegm

Indications: Phlegm damp cough and bronchitis

Ingredients: Exocarpium Rubrum Citri Reticulatae (*Ju Hong*), 12g, Semen Pruni Armeniacae (*Xing Ren*), 6g, Semen Oryzae Sativae (*i.e.*, Polished Rice, *Jing Mi*), 50g

Method of preparation & administration: First decoct the first 2 ingredients in water, remove the dregs, and reserve the liquid. Make porridge out of the rice using this liquid and eat 1-2 times per day.

Two Aged (Ingredients) & Two Seeds Congee
(Er Chen Er Ren Zhou)

Functions: Eliminates dampness and transforms phlegm

Indications: Phlegm damp cough and bronchitis

Ingredients: Pericarpium Citri Reticulatae (*Chen Pi*), 9g, Rhizoma Pinelliae Ternatae (*Ban Xia*), 6g, Sclerotium Poriae Cocos (*Fu Ling*), 12g, Semen Coicis Lachryma-jobi (*Yi Yi Ren*), 12g, Semen Benincasae Hispidae (*Dong Gua Ren*), 15g, Semen Oryzae Sativae (*i.e.*, Polished Rice, *Jing Mi*), 100g

Method of preparation & administration: First decoct the first 5 ingredients in water, remove the dregs, and reserve the liquid. Then make the rice into porridge using this liquid. Take 2 times per day.

Eriobotrya Flower Congee
(Pi Pa Hua Zhou)

Functions: Warms the lungs and stops coughing, transforms phlegm and levels panting (*i.e.*, asthma)

Indications: Chronic bronchitis, cough, cough with phlegm, qi panting (*i.e.*, asthma)

Ingredients: Dry Flos Eriobotryae Japonicae (*Gan Pi Pa Hua*), 30g, Semen Oryzae Sativae (*i.e.*, Polished Rice, *Jing Mi*), 50g

Method of preparation & administration: Add water and cook into porridge as usual and eat occasionally.

Eriobotrya Leaf Congee
(Pi Pa Ye Zhou)

Functions: Transforms phlegm and stops coughing, harmonizes the stomach and downbears counterflow

Indications: Lung heat cough, coughing and vomiting a yellow colored pussy phlegm and coughing blood, stomach heat vomiting and hiccup, wind heat common cold, acute bronchitis, pneumonia, lung abscess, acute gastritis

Ingredients: Folium Eriobotryae Japonicae (*Pi Pa Ye*), 15g, Semen Oryzae Sativae (*i.e.*, Polished Rice, *Jing Mi*), 100g, Granulated Sugar (*Bing Tang*), a small amount

Method of preparation & administration: First decoct the Eriobotrya leaves in 200ml of water down to 100ml, remove the dregs, and reserve the liquid. Add this liquid plus 600ml of water to the rice and sugar and cook into porridge. Eat warm each day in the morning and evening.

Phragmites & Fritillaria Congee
(*Lu Gen Chuan Bei Zhou*)

Functions: Clears heat and transforms phlegm

Indications: Phlegm heat cough and bronchitis

Ingredients: Rhizoma Phragmitis Communis (*Lu Gen*), 45g, Bulbus Fritillariae Cirrhosae (*Chuan Bei Mu*), 9g, Caulis In Taeniis Bambusae (*Zhu Ru*), 12g, Semen Oryzae Sativae (*i.e.*, Polished Rice, *Jing Mi*), 100g, Granulated Sugar (*Bing Tang*), 15g

Method of preparation & administration: First decoct the first 3 ingredients in water, remove the dregs, and reserve the liquid. Then make porridge from the rice using this liquid and a suitable amount of water. Put in the sugar at the end of the cooking and eat 2 times per day.

Mulberry Bark Congee
(*Sang Bai Pi Zhou*)

Functions: Drains the lungs and levels panting (*i.e.*, asthma), disinhibits urination and disperses swelling

Indications: Lung heat cough, panting and counterflow with excessive phlegm or superficial edema of the face and eyes, inhibited urination, pediatric bronchitis, diabetes mellitus, etc.

Ingredients: Cortex Radicis Mori Albi (*Sang Bai Pi*), 15g, Semen Oryzae Sativae (*i.e.*, Polished Rice, *Jing Mi*), 50g, Granulated Sugar (*Bing Tang*), a suitable amount

Method of preparation & administration: First decoct the mulberry bark in 200ml of water down to 100ml, remove the dregs, and reserve the liquid. Add this and 400ml more water to the rice and sugar and cook into porridge. Eat warm 2 times per day.

Contraindications: Do not use for lung cold cough or wind cold common cold cough.

Chinese Green Olive Congee
(*Qing Guo Zhou*)

Functions: Clears heat and resolves toxins, engenders fluids and stops thirst, clears the lungs and disinhibits the throat

Indications: Upper respiratory infections, cough, cough with phlegm, swollen, painful, inflamed throat

Ingredients: Fructus Canarii Pimelae (*Qing Guo*), 10 pieces, Semen Oryzae Sativae (*i.e.*, Polished Rice, *Da Mi*), 50g

Method of preparation & administration: First boil the Chinese olives 2 times, throwing out the water until it becomes clear. Then add the rice and Chinese olives together and cook into porridge as usual.

Dry Preserved Cabbage Congee
(*Gan Dong Cai Zhou*)

Functions: Nourishes yin, fortifies the spleen, transforms phlegm, descends the qi

Indications: Lung heat cough, laryngitis

Ingredients: Dry Preserved Cabbage (*Gan Dong Cai*), 50g, Semen Oryzae Sativae (*i.e.*, Polished Rice, *Da Mi*), 50g

Method of preparation & administration: Cook into porridge as usual. Use a small amount of peanut oil (*Hua Sheng You*) to flavor and eat.

Aduki Bean, Lily Bulb & Apricot Seed Congee
(*Chi Xiao Dou Bai He Xing Ren Zhou*)

Functions: Moistens the lungs and stops cough, eliminates phlegm and disinhibits dampness

Indications: Lung dryness with damp phlegm obstructing internally, qi not engendering fluids resulting in cough, panting, dry mouth, excessive phlegm, and inhibited urination

Ingredients: Semen Phaseoli Calcarati (*i.e.*, Aduki Beans, *Chi Xiao Dou*), 60g, Bulbus Lilii (*Bai He*), 10g, Semen Pruni Armeniacae (*Xing Ren*), 6g, White Sugar (*Bai Tang*), a suitable amount

Method of preparation & administration: First cook the aduki beans as usual. Then add the lily bulbs and apricot seeds and continue cooking. Add sugar to taste and eat.

Chinese Yam Congee
(*Shan Yao Zhou*)

Functions: Supplements the spleen and stops diarrhea, supplements the kidneys and restrains and contains

Indications: Taxation cough and panting (*i.e.*, asthma), spleen vacuity diarrhea, and other pathoconditions associated with weakness, vacuity, and detriment

Ingredients: Fresh Radix Dioscoreae Oppositae (*Sheng Huai Shan Yao*), 30g, White Sugar (*Bai Tang*), a small amount

Method of preparation & administration: Chop up the Chinese yam into small pieces and add to cool water. Cook and stir bringing to a boil 2-3 times. Add a small amount of white sugar to taste and eat.

Bamboo Juice Congee
(Zhu Li Zhou)

Functions: Clears heat, sweeps away phlegm, settles fright

Indications: Wind heat, phlegm fire, lung heat cough with excessive phlegm which is yellow in color

Ingredients: Succus Bambusae (*i.e.*, Bamboo Juice, *Zhu Li*), 30g, Semen Oryzae Sativae (*i.e.*, Polished Rice, *Jing Mi*), 100g

Method of preparation & administration: First cook the rice into porridge. While still hot, add the bamboo juice and stir. Eat as one wishes.

Lycium Root Bark Congee
(Di Gu Pi Zhou)

Functions: Clears heat and enriches yin, cools the blood and recedes fever, stops bleeding

Indications: Steaming bone and tidal fever, epistaxis, hemoptysis, hematuria, lung heat cough, high blood pressure, tuberculosis, diabetes mellitus

Ingredients: Cortex Radicis Lycii (*Di Gu Pi*), 30g, Semen Oryzae Sativae (*i.e.*, Polished Rice, *Jing Mi*), 50g, Granulated Sugar (*Bing Tang*), a suitable amount

Method of preparation & administration: First decoct the Cortex Radicis Lycii in water, remove the dregs, and reserve 100ml of liquid. Add this liquid plus 400ml more water to the rice and sugar and cook into porridge as usual. Eat warm 2 times per day.

Butter & Honey Congee
(*Su Mi Zhou*)

Functions: Supplements the five viscera, boosts qi and blood, engenders fluids, and moistens dryness

Indications: Bodily weakness, emaciation, vacuity taxation low-grade fever, lung atony, lung dryness, cough, vomiting blood, dry, withered, coarse skin, dry, knotted, difficult stools

Ingredients: Butter (*Su You*), 30g, Honey (*Mi Tang*), 30g, Semen Oryzae Sativae (*i.e.*, Polished Rice, *Jing Mi*), 100g

Method of preparation & administration: Make porridge out of the rice and 800ml of water. Then add the butter and honey to the porridge and cook until it thickens. Eat warm 2 times per day in the morning and evening. Three days equal 1 course of treatment.

Wood Ear Congee
(*Mu Er Zhou*)

Functions: Enriches yin and moistens the lungs

Indications: Lung yin vacuity taxation cough, coughing blood, qi panting (*i.e.*, asthma), and other such conditions

Ingredients: Black Fructificatio Tremellae (*Hei Mu Er*), 5g, Fructus Zizyphi Jujubae (*Da Zao*), 5 pieces, Semen Oryzae Sativae (*i.e.*, Polished Rice, *Jing Mi*), 100g, Granulated Sugar (*Bing Tang*), a suitable amount

Method of preparation & administration: Soak the black wood ears in warm water to soften. Then cook into porridge with the rice and jujubes. Add sugar to taste and eat on a regular basis.

Pearl & Jade Two Treasures Congee
(*Zhen Yu Er Bao Zhou*)

Functions: Enriches and nourishes the spleen and lungs, stops coughing and dispels phlegm

Indications: Spleen/lung yin deficiency, reduced appetite, vacuity taxation cough

Ingredients: Fresh Radix Dioscoreae Oppositae (*Sheng Shan Yao*), 60g, raw Semen Coicis Lachryma-jobi (*Sheng Yi Mi*), 60g, Persimmon Frost (*Shi Shuang*), 24g

Method of preparation & administration: Grind the Dioscorea and Coix into small pieces and cook into porridge. Mix in the persimmon frost and eat on a regular basis.

Pork Lung Congee
(*Zhu Fei Zhou*)

Functions: Supplements the lungs and stops cough

Indications: Enduring cough due to lung qi vacuity, excessive phlegm, hemoptysis, and other such conditions

Ingredients: Pork Lung (*Zhu Fei*), 500g, Semen Coicis Lachryma-jobi (*Yi Yi Ren*), 50g, Semen Oryzae Sativae (*i.e.*, Polished Rice, *Da Mi*), 100g, Herba Allii Fistulosi (*i.e.*, Scallion, *Cong*), a suitable amount, Fresh Rhizoma Zingiberis (*i.e.*, Fresh Ginger, *Sheng Jiang*), a suitable amount, Salt (*Yan*), a suitable amount, Cooking Wine (*Liao Jiu*), a suitable amount

Method of preparation & administration: Wash the pork lungs, put in water and some cooking wine, and bring to a boil 7 times. Then cut the lungs into pieces. Add to the rice and Coix and cook into porridge, adding the scallions, ginger, and salt near the end of cooking. Eat frequently.

Glutinous Rice, Ginseng & Ophiopogon Congee
(Nuo Mi Shen Dong Zhou)

Functions: Boosts the qi and enriches yin, settles cough and expels phlegm

Indications: Cough, chronic bronchitis, heart palpitations, lack of strength, etc.

Ingredients: Semen Oryzae Glutinosae (*i.e.*, Glutinous Rice, *Nuo Mi*), 100g, Tuber Ophiopogonis Japonicae (*Mai Men Dong*), 5g, Radix Panacis Ginseng (*Ren Shen*), 1.5g, Radix Glycyrrhizae (*Gan Cao*), 1.5g, Fructus Zizyphi Jujubae (*Hong Zao*), 3 pieces, Honey (*Mi Tang*), a suitable amount

Method of preparation & administration: First decoct the first 4 ingredients, remove the dregs, and reserve the liquid. Then cook the rice into porridge, add this medicinal liquid, and continue cooking till done. Add honey to taste and eat.

Glehnia Congee
(Sha Shen Zhou)

Functions: Moistens the lungs and nourishes the stomach, nourishes yin and clears heat, dispels phlegm and stops coughing

Indications: Lung heat and dryness cough, dry cough without phlegm, enduring cough, stomach yin insufficiency, scant fluids, dry mouth, a scant tongue coating

Ingredients: Radix Glehniae Littoralis (*Bei Sha Shen*), 15g, Semen Oryzae Sativae (*i.e.*, Polished Rice, *Da Mi*), 50g, Granulated Sugar (*Bing Tang*), a suitable amount

Method of preparation & administration: Cook the rice and sugar into porridge as usual. Powder the Glehnia and add to the porridge. Cook a few minutes more and eat 1 time each morning and evening. Five to 7 days equal 1 course of treatment.

Trichosanthes Root Congee
(Tian Hua Fen Zhou)

Functions: Clears heat and engenders fluids, disperses swelling and expels pus

Indications: Lung heat and dryness cough, damaged fluids due to febrile disease, wasting and thirsting, ulcers and toxic swellings

Ingredients: Radix Trichosanthis Kirlowii (*Tian Hua Fen*), 30g, Semen Oryzae Sativae (*i.e.*, Polished Rice, *Jing Mi*), 50g

Method of preparation & administration: Soak the Trichosanthes root for 2 hours in warm water. Then add 200ml of water and decoct down to 100ml, remove the dregs, and reserve the liquid. Add 400ml of water to the rice plus this reserved liquid and cook into porridge. Take 2-3 times per day after allowing to cool.

Astragalus & Pork Lung Congee
(Huang Qi Zhu Fei Zhou)

Functions: Supplements the lungs, boosts the qi, and enriches yin

Indications: Lung qi and yin vacuity enduring cough and bronchitis

Ingredients: Pork Lung (*Zhu Fei*), 100g, Radix Astragali Membranacei (*Huang Qi*), 30g, Semen Oryzae Sativae (*i.e.*, Polished Rice, *Jing Mi*), 100g, Bulbus Allii Fistulosi (*i.e.*, Scallion, *Cong Bai*), a suitable amount, fresh Rhizoma Zingiberis (*i.e.*, Fresh Ginger, *Sheng Jiang*), a suitable amount, Salt (*Yan*), a suitable amount

Method of preparation & administration: First wash the pork lung and boil in a suitable amount of water. When cooked, chop into pieces. Then decoct the Astragalus, remove the dregs, and reserve the liquid.

Cook the rice and chopped pork lung in this liquid and cook into porridge. Add scallion, ginger, and salt to taste. Eat in 2 divided doses per day.

Polygonatum Congee
(Huang Jing Zhou)

Functions: Moistens the lungs, enriches yin, and supplements the spleen

Indications: Lung yin insufficiency dry cough without phlegm, lung consumption, hemoptysis, spleen/stomach vacuity weakness, bodily vacuity, scant appetite, fatigue, lack of strength

Ingredients: Dry Rhizoma Polygonati (*Gan Huang Jing*), 15g, Semen Oryzae Sativae (*i.e.*, Polished Rice, *Da Mi*), 50g, Pericarpium Citri Reticulatae (*Chen Pi*), 2g, Granulated Sugar (*Bing Tang*), a suitable amount

Method of preparation & administration: First cook the rice into porridge. Add the finely powdered orange peel. Cut up the P-olygonatum finely and add those slices to the porridge as well and cook for some time longer. Eat warm each morning and evening.

Lily Bulb, Fragrant Solomon's Seal & Two Winters Congee (*Bai Yu Er Dong Zhou*)

Functions: Supplements the lungs and kidneys and enriches yin

Indications: Chronic cough and bronchitis due to lung/kidney yin vacuity

Ingredients: Bulbus Lilii (*Bai He*), 30g, Rhizoma Polygonati Odorati (*Yu Zhu*), 12g, Tuber Asparagi Cochinensis (*Tian Men Dong*), 12g, Tuber Ophiopogonis Japonicae (*Mai Men Dong*), 12g, Semen Oryzae Sativae (*i.e.*, Polished Rice, *Jing Mi*), 100g, Honey (*Mi Tang*), 15g

Method of preparation & administration: First decoct the first 4 ingredients in water, remove the dregs, and reserve the liquid. Then cook the rice into a porridge using this liquid. Add the honey at the end. Eat in 2 divided doses per day.

Four Seeds & Egg Congee
(*Si Ren Ji Zi Zhou*)

Functions: Supplements the lungs and kidneys and enriches yin

Indications: Chronic cough and bronchitis due to lung/kidney yin vacuity

Ingredients: Semen Gingkonis Bilobae (*Bai Guo*), 1 part, Sweet Semen Pruni Armeniacae (*Gan Xing Ren*), 1 part, Semen Juglandis Regiae (*i.e.*, Walnut, *Hu Tao Ren*), 2 parts, Semen Arachidis (*i.e.*, Peanut, *Hua Sheng Ren*), 2 parts, Egg (*Ji Zi*), 1

Method of preparation & administration: Grind the first 4 ingredients into powder and mix thoroughly. Cook 20g of this powder with 1 egg and eat every morning for 1/2 year continuously.

5
Pneumonia (*Fei Yan*)

Phragmites & Bamboo Juice Congee
(*Lu Gen Zhu Li Zhou*)

Functions: Clears replete heat from the lungs

Indications: Lung heat obstruction and exuberance pneumonia

Ingredients: Rhizoma Phragmitis Communis (*Lu Gen*), 60g, Semen Oryzae Sativae (*i.e.*, Polished Rice, *Jing Mi*), 50g, Succus Bambusae (*Zhu Li*), 30g, Granulated Sugar (*Bing Tang*), 15g

Method of preparation & administration: First decoct the Phragmites, remove the dregs, and reserve the liquid. Then cook the rice in this liquid into porridge. When the porridge is cooked, add the bamboo juice and sugar and cook for a short time more. Eat 1-2 times per day as an adjunctive treatment.

Compound Houttuynia Congee
(*Fu Fang Yu Xing Cao Zhou*)

Functions: Clears replete heat from the lungs

Indications: Lung heat obstruction and exuberance pneumonia

Ingredients: Herba Houttuyniae Cordatae (*Yu Xing Cao*), 30g, Flos Lonicerae Japonicae (*Yin Hua*), 30g, Rhizoma Phragmitis Communis (*Lu Gen*), 30g, raw Gypsum Fibrosum (*Sheng Shi Gao*), Caulis In Taeniis Bambusae (*Zhu Ru*), 9g, Semen Oryzae Sativae (*i.e.*, Polished Rice, *Jing Mi*), 100g, Granulated Sugar (*Bing Tang*), 30g

Method of preparation & administration: Decoct the first 5 ingredients in water, remove the dregs, and reserve the liquid. Then cook the rice into porridge using this liquid plus some additional water. Add the sugar and continue cooking a few minutes more. Eat 2 times per day.

6
Coughing & Panting (*i.e.*, Asthma)
(*Ke Chuan*)

Ephedra & Dry Ginger Congee
(*Ma Huang Gan Jiang Zhou*)

Functions: Relieves the exterior and scatters cold, diffuses the lungs and levels panting

Indications: Wind cold panting (*i.e.*, asthma)

Ingredients: Herba Ephedrae (*Ma Huang*), 6g, dry Rhizoma Zingiberis (*Gan Jiang*), 6g, Radix Glycyrrhizae (*Gan Cao*), 3g, Semen Oryzae

Sativae (*i.e.*, Polished Rice, *Jing Mi*), 100g, Bulbus Allii Fistulosi (*i.e.*, Scallion, *Cong Bai*), 3g

Method of preparation & administration: Decoct the first 3 ingredients in water, remove the dregs, and reserve the liquid. Make the rice into porridge using this liquid. When the porridge is cooked, sprinkle the chopped scallion on the top and eat 2 times per day as an adjunctive treatment for asthma.

Millet & Lamb Fetus Congee
(*Xiao Mi Yang Tai Zhou*)

Functions: Supplements the kidneys and boosts the qi, stops coughing and promotes absorption of the qi

Indications: Lack of strength of the low back and knees, chronic cough and qi panting (*i.e.*, asthma) with movement leading to an asthmatic attack

Ingredients: Semen Setariae Italicae (*i.e.*, Millet, *Xiao Mi*), Lamb Fetus (*Yang Tai*), 1 piece

Method of preparation & administration: First cook the lamb fetus until half-cooked. Then add the millet and make into porridge. Eat the porridge with the meat in it 2 times each day.

Eye-Brightening Tea Congee
(*Qing Ming Cha Zhou*)

Functions: Warms the lungs and loosens the chest, transforms phlegm and stops coughing

Indications: Enduring cough with excessive phlegm, panting and qi counterflow, taxation cough, lung decline

Ingredients: Herba Gnaphalii Multicepsis (*Qing Ming Cha*, a.k.a. *Shu Chu Cao*), 15g, Semen Oryzae Sativae (*i.e.*, Polished Rice, *Jing Mi*), 50g

Method of preparation & administration: First decoct the Gnaphalium Multiceps, remove the dregs, and reserve the liquid. Then using this liquid, cook the rice into porridge. Eat on an empty stomach.

Apricot Seed Congee
(Xing Ren Zhou)

Functions: Clears and drains lung heat, stops cough and levels panting, descends the qi and loosens the chest

Indications: Lung vacuity hurried breathing, cough, chest fullness with excessive phlegm, etc.

Ingredients: Semen Pruni Armeniacae (*Xing Ren*), 10g, Radix Codonopsis Pilosulae (*Dang Shen*), 30g, Cortex Radicis Mori (*Sang Bai Pi*), 10g, fresh Rhizoma Zingiberis (*i.e.*, Fresh Ginger, *Sheng Jiang*), 6g, Fructus Ziziphi Jujubae (*Da Zao*), 7 pieces, Cow's Milk (*Niu Nai*), 200ml, Semen Oryzae Sativae (*i.e.*, Polished Rice, *Jing Mi*), 100g

Method of preparation & administration: First soak the apricot seeds and remove the skin and tips. Then grind into powder and place in the cow's milk, cook and stir. Then decoct the Codonopsis, Morus, ginger, and jujubes and remove the dregs. Combine the resulting decoction with the porridge and cook some more, always stirring. Finally take as much as one wishes on an empty stomach.

Peach Seed Congee
(Tao Ren Zhou)

Functions: Supplements the lungs and kidneys, harmonizes the stomach and regulates the center

Indications: Cough, chest fullness, qi panting (*i.e.*, asthma), bronchitis

Ingredients: Semen Pruni Persicae (*Tao Ren*), 10g, Semen Oryzae Sativae (*i.e.*, Polished Rice, *Jing Mi*), 100g

Method of preparation & administration: First soak the peach seeds in water to remove the outer skin. Then grind into a mash, cook into porridge with the rice, and eat.

Walnut Congee
(Hu Tao Zhou)

Functions: Supplements the kidneys and strengthens the low back and knees, boosts the lungs and stabilizes panting (*i.e.*, asthma) and coughing

Indications: Lung/kidney dual vacuity, shortness of breath, panting and coughing, low back and knee soreness and weakness, lack of strength of the lower legs and feet, constipation in the elderly, tuberculosis, low back muscles taxation detriment, poor nutrition, bodily vacuity weakness, etc.

Ingredients: Semen Juglandis Regiae (*i.e.*, Walnuts, *Hu Tao Ren*), 50g, Semen Oryzae Sativae (*i.e.*, Polished Rice, *Jing Mi*), 50g

Method of preparation & administration: First remove the shells and skin of the walnuts and pound into a mash. Add water to the rice and cook into porridge. After the porridge is cooked, add the walnut mash and stir in thoroughly. Skim any oil off the top of the porridge and eat warm 1 time each morning and evening.

Cordyceps Congee
(Chong Cao Zhou)

Functions: Boosts the lungs, supplements the kidneys, and enriches yin, stops panting (*i.e.*, asthma)

Indications: Lung yin insufficiency, vacuity panting and taxation cough, hemoptysis, dry phlegm, spontaneous sweating, night sweats, impotence, spermatorrhea, low back and knee aching and pain, bodily weakness and enduring vacuity in the aftermath of disease

Ingredients: Powdered Cordyceps Sinensis (*Dong Chong Xia Cao Fen*), 6g, powdered Rhizoma Bletillae Striatae (*Bai Ji Fen*), 6g, Semen

Oryzae Sativae (*i.e.*, Polished Rice, *Da Mi*), 50g, Granulated Sugar (*Bing Tang*), a suitable amount

Method of preparation & administration: First cook the rice and sugar into porridge as usual. After the rice is cooked, add the powdered Cordyceps and Bletilla, mix thoroughly, and cook a short time more. Eat warm 2 times per day. Five to 7 days equal 1 course of treatment.

7
Pulmonary Tuberculosis (*Fei Jie He*)

Brown Rice Congee
(*Cao Jing Mi Zhou*)

Functions: Clears heat, disinhibits dampness, expels pus

Indications: Pulmonary tuberculosis, anemia

Ingredients: Brown Rice (*Cao Mi*), 100g, Semen Coicis Lachryma-jobi (*Yi Mi Ren*), 50g, Fructus Zizyphi Jujubae (*Hong Zao*), 8 pieces

Method of preparation & administration: Cook the above two grains into porridge, add the jujubes, and eat 1 time in the morning and evening.

Lily Bulb Porridge
(*Bai He Zhou*)

Functions: Moistens the lungs and stops coughing, clears the heart and quiets the spirit

Indications: Enduring cough due to lung consumption, cough mixed with phlegm, vacuity vexation, palpitations, emotional instability

Ingredients: Bulbus Lilii (*Bai He*), 60g, Semen Oryzae Sativae (*i.e.*, Polished Rice, *Da Mi*), 250g, White Sugar (*Bai Tang*), 100g

Method of preparation & administration: Cook the rice and lily bulbs together into porridge. Then add sugar and eat warm 3-5 times per day.

Bletilla, Rice & Garlic Congee
(Bai Ji Mi Suan Zhou)

Functions: Stops bleeding, especially from the lungs

Indications: Hemoptysis due to externally invading evils

Ingredients: Rhizoma Bletillae Striatae (*Bai Ji*), 5g, Garlic (with purplish skins, *Zi Pi Da Suan*), 30g, Polished Rice, 60g

Method of preparation & administration: First blanch the garlic and remove their skins. Then cook the rice and Bletilla into porridge as usual. Add the garlic and continue cooking till done. Eat frequently in the morning and evening.

8
Meningitis (Nao Mao Yan)

Lotus Flower Congee
(Lian Hua Zhou)

Functions: Clears the heart, cools the blood, resolves toxins

Indications: Loss of consciousness due to hot toxins, vexatious thirst and desire for cold drinks or pediatric fright convulsions, possible heart fire hyperactivity and exuberance, vexation and agitation, insomnia, etc.

Ingredients: Flos Nelumbinis Nuciferae (*Lian Hua*), 6g, Semen Oryzae Sativae (*i.e.*, Polished Rice, *Jing Mi*), 50g

Method of preparation & administration: Pick the lotus flowers in the 6-7th (Chinese) months and dry in the shade. Then grind into a powder and store for use. First cook the rice into porridge. Then add the lotus flowers and continue cooking, stirring the powder into the porridge completely. Eat on an empty stomach.

9
Indigestion (*Xiao Hua Bu Liang*)

Barley Congee
(*Da Mai Mi Zhou*)

Functions: Loosens the center and descends the qi, disinhibits urination

Indications: Middle burner qi obstruction, indigestion, abdominal distention, inhibited urination

Ingredients: Fructus Hordei Vulgaris (*i.e.*, Barley, *Da Mai Mi*), 50g, Red Sugar (*i.e.*, Brown Sugar, *Hong Tang*), a suitable amount.

Method of preparation & administration: Cook the barley in water to make into porridge.

Contraindications: Do not eat in case of spleen/stomach qi vacuity or spleen/stomach smoldering heat.

Medicated Leaven Congee
(*Qu Mi Zhou*)

Functions: Disperses and transforms grain foods, fortifies the spleen and harmonizes the stomach

Indications: Damage by food, accumulations and stagnation, external invasion, indigestion, diarrhea

Ingredients: Massa Medica Fermentata (*Shen Qu*), 15g, Semen Oryzae Sativae (*i.e.*, Polished Rice, *Jing Mi*), 100g

Method of preparation & administration: First grind the Medicated Leaven into powder. Add 200ml of water and decoct down to 100ml. Remove the dregs and reserve the liquid. Add this plus 600ml of water to the rice and cook into porridge. Eat warm each day in the morning and evening.

Plum Flower Congee
(Mei Hua Zhou)

Functions: Courses the liver and resolves depression, fortifies the spleen and opens the stomach

Indications: Liver/stomach qi pain, plum pit qi, chest oppression, lack of relaxation, diminished appetite

Ingredients: Semen Oryzae Sativae (*i.e.*, Polished Rice, *Jing Mi*), 100g, White Sugar (*Bai Tang*), a small amount, Flos Pruni (*Mei Hua*), 5g

Method of preparation & administration: Cook the rice into porridge as usual. Add the plum flowers and bring back to a boil. Then add sugar to taste and eat warm every morning and evening. Three to 5 days equal 1 course of treatment.

Lamb & Sorghum Congee
(Yang Rou Shu Mi Zhou)

Functions: Opens the stomach and fortifies the strength

Indications: Spleen/stomach vacuity weakness leading to indigestion, abdominal cramping pain, etc.

Ingredients: Lamb (*Yang Rou*), 100g, Semen Panici Miliaci (*i.e.*, husked Sorghum, *Shu Mi*), 100g, Salt (*Yan Sha*) to taste

Method of preparation & administration: Cut the lamb into pieces, add to the sorghum, cook into porridge, and eat.

Barbarian Radish (I.e., Carrot) Congee
(Hu Luo Bo Zhou)

Functions: Supplements the center and boosts the qi, disperses distention and transforms stagnation

Indications: Abdominal distention and food stagnation

Ingredients: Radix Dauci Caroti (*i.e.*, Carrot, *Hu Luo Bo*), 500g, Semen Oryzae Sativae (*i.e.*, Polished Rice, *Jing Mi*), 100g, Red Sugar (*i.e.*, Brown Sugar, *Hong Tang*), a suitable amount

Method of preparation & administration: Cut the carrot into small pieces and cook with the rice in water into porridge. Add the brown sugar and eat warm.

Jujube & Millet Congee
(*Xiao Zao Su Mi Zhou*)

Functions: Nourishes the intestines and stomach, clears vacuity heat

Indications: Indigestion due to fluid dryness and vacuity heat, also postpartum vacuity weakness

Ingredients: Semen Setariae Italicae (*i.e.*, Millet, *Su Mi*), 100g, small Fructus Zizyphi Jujubae (*Xiao Zao*), 50g, Red Sugar (*i.e.*, Brown Sugar, *Hong Tang*), 50g

Method of preparation & administration: Cook the above ingredients into porridge and eat occasionally with brown sugar.

Osmanthus Flower Congee
(*Gui Hua Zhou*)

Functions: Arouses the spleen and delights the spirit

Indications: Diseases due to spleen dampness, phlegm rheum cough and panting, stomach mouth not open, intestinal wind bloody dysentery, toothache, bad breath, etc.

Ingredients: Flos Osmanthi Fragrantis (*Gui Hua*, dried in the shade), 3g, Semen Oryzae Sativae (*i.e.*, Polished Rice, *Jing Mi*), 50g, Red Sugar (*i.e.*, Brown Sugar, *Hong Tang*), a small amount

Method of preparation: Cook the osmanthus flowers and rice together into porridge. Add the brown sugar and eat.

10
Vomiting & Hiccup (*Ou Tu, E Ni*)

Buddha's Hand Flower Congee
(*Fo Shou Hua Zhou*)

Functions: Courses the liver and harmonizes the stomach, diffuses the center and transforms turbidity

Indications: Liver depression/qi stagnation, stomach qi not relaxed, upward counterflow, hiccup, torpid intake

Ingredients: Dry Flos Citri Sacrodactyli (*Gan Fo Shou Hua*), 30g, Semen Oryzae Sativae (*i.e.*, Polished Rice, *Jing Mi*), 50g

Method of preparation & administration: Add water and make into porridge as usual. Take 1 time each morning and evening.

Phragmites & Mung Bean Congee
(*Lu Gen Lu Dou Zhou*)

Functions: Stops vomiting, disinhibits urination

Indications: Damp heat vomiting and vexatious thirst due to febrile disease, red, astringent urination. Also resolves fish and crab toxins.

Ingredients: Semen Phaseoli Mungonis (*i.e.*, Mung Beans, *Lu Dou*), 100g, Rhizoma Phragmitis Communis (*Lu Gen*), 100g, fresh Rhizoma Zingiberis (*i.e.*, Fresh Ginger, *Sheng Jiang*), 10g, Folium Perillae Frutescentis (*Zi Su Ye*), 15g

Method of preparation & administration: First decoct the Phragmites, ginger, and Perilla leaves. Remove the dregs and reserve the liquid. Add this liquid to the mung beans and cook into porridge. Eat as one pleases.

Bamboo Shavings Congee
(Zhu Ru Zhou)

Functions: Clears heat from the stomach and harmonizes the middle, eliminates vexation and stops vomiting

Indications: Lung and stomach heat, vomiting during pregnancy, postpartum vexation and bodily weakness in the aftermath of disease, vacuity heat vexatious thirst

Ingredients: Caulis In Taeniis Bambusae (*Zhu Ru*), 15g, Semen Oryzae Sativae (*i.e.*, Polished Rice, *Jing Mi*), 50g, fresh Rhizoma Zingiberis (*i.e.*, Fresh Ginger, *i.e.*, Fresh Ginger, *Sheng Jiang*), 2 slices

Method of preparation and administration: First decoct the bamboo shavings in water, remove the dregs, and reserve 100ml of this liquid. Then make porridge from the rice and 400ml of water. When the porridge is cooked, add the medicinal liquid and the ginger and bring back to a boil 1 time. Eat warm 2 times per day.

Contraindications: Do not use for stomach cold vomiting.

Swordbean Congee
(Dao Dou Zhou)

Functions: Warms the center and boosts the qi, descends the qi and stops hiccup

Indications: Vacuity cold stomach pain, hiccup, vomiting, and other such conditions

Ingredients: Semen Canavalliae Ensiformis (*Dao Dou*), 15g, Semen Oryzae Sativae (*i.e.*, Polished Rice, *Jing Mi*), 50g, fresh Rhizoma Zingiberis (*i.e.*, Fresh Ginger, *Sheng Jiang*), 2 slices

Method of preparation & administration: Cook into porridge as usual and eat warm each day in the morning and evening.

Dry Ginger Congee
(*Gan Jiang Zhou*)

Functions: Fortifies the stomach and stops vomiting, warms the center and scatters cold

Indications: Stomach cold vomiting, spleen cold diarrhea (*i.e.*, chronic gastritis, chronic colitis, indigestion), lung cold cough (*i.e.*, chronic bronchitis)

Ingredients: Powdered Dry Rhizoma Zingiberis (*Gan Jiang Fen*), 5g, Semen Oryzae Sativae (*i.e.*, Polished Rice, *Da Mi*), 100g

Method of preparation & administration: Cook the rice, ginger powder, and water into porridge as usual. Eat each morning on an empty stomach.

Fennel Congee
(*Hui Xiang Zhou*)

Functions: Harmonizes the stomach, moves the qi, scatters cold, and stops pain

Indications: Small intestine *shan* qi, epigastric and abdominal qi distention, testicular swelling, distention, and heaviness, stomach cold vomiting, diminished appetite, chronic gastritis

Ingredients: Fructus Feoniculi Vulgaris (*i.e.*, Fennel, *Xiao Hui Xiang*), 30g, Semen Oryzae Sativae (*i.e.*, Polished Rice, *Jing Mi*), 50g, Red Sugar (*i.e.*, Brown Sugar, *Hong Tang*), a suitable amount

Method of preparation & administration: First stir-fry the fennel till it turns a burnt yellow. Then grind it into a fine powder and store for use. This amount equals enough for 1 course of treatment. Next cook the rice in water into porridge as usual. Add 5-6g of fennel powder and the sugar and continue cooking for some time more. Eat warm, 1 time per day, each evening before going to bed. Five days equal 1 course of treatment.

Chinese Yam & Pinellia Congee
(Shan Yao Ban Xia Zhou)

Functions: Fortifies the spleen and harmonizes the stomach, downbears counterflow and stops vomiting

Indications: Spleen/stomach vacuity weakness leading to qi counterflow and upward thrusting

Ingredients: Fresh Radix Dioscoreae Oppositae (*Sheng Shan Yao*), 30g, Rhizoma Pinelliae Ternatae (*Qing Ban Xia*), 30g, White Sugar (*Bai Tang*), a suitable amount

Method of preparation & administration: Grind the Dioscorea into a fine powder. Wash the Pinellia in slightly warm water several times. Then decoct the Pinellia, remove the dregs, and reserve the liquid. Add the Dioscorea powder and bring to a boil 3 times, thus making it into a porridge. Add the sugar and eat at no fixed times.

Sparrow Congee
(Ma Que Zhou)

Functions: Stops hiccup in the elderly

Indications: Hiccup in the elderly. It also improves impotence due to lack of erection.

Ingredients: Passer Montanus Saturatus (*i.e.*, Sparrow, *Ma Que*), 5 pieces, Semen Oryzae Sativae (*i.e.*, Polished Rice, *Da Mi*), 50g, Salt (*Yan Sha*), to taste

Method of preparation & administration: First remove the skin and guts of the sparrows. Then add to the rice and cook into porridge. Add salt to taste and eat immediately.

11
Stomach Pain (*Wei Tong*)

Galangal & Rice Congee
(*Liang Jiang Jing Mi Zhou*)

Functions: Expels cold and disperses accumulations and gatherings

Indications: Chilly pain in the heart and abdomen, accumulations and gatherings, collection of rheum

Ingredients: Rhizoma Alpiniae Officinari (*Gao Liang Jiang*), 15g, Semen Oryzae Sativae (*i.e.*, Polished Rice, *Jing Mi*), 100g

Method of preparation & administration: First decoct the galangal, remove the dregs, and reserve the liquid. Add this to the rice, cook into porridge, and eat.

Galangal & Cyperus Congee
(*Liang Fu Zhou*)

Functions: Warms the center and rectifies the qi

Indications: Stomach cold and/or qi stagnation epigastric pain

Ingredients: Rhizoma Alpiniae Officinari (*Liang Jiang*), 9g, Rhizoma Cyperi Rotundi (*Xiang Fu*), 9g, Semen Oryzae Sativae (*i.e.*, Polished Rice, *Jing Mi*), 100g

Method of preparation & administration: Decoct the first 2 ingredients in water, remove the dregs, and reserve the liquid. Use this liquid to make porridge out of the rice and eat 2 times per day.

Move the Qi & Fortify the Stomach Congee
(*Xing Qi Jian Wei Zhou*)

Functions: Rectifies the qi and harmonizes the stomach

Indications: Qi stagnation epigastric pain

Ingredients: Fructus Amomi (*Sha Ren*), 3g, Pericarpium Citri Reticulatae (*Chen Pi*), 6g, Fructus Citri Seu Ponciri (*Zhi Qiao*), 6g, Fructus Citri Sacrodactylis (*Fo Shou*), 6g, Semen Oryzae Sativae (*i.e.*, Polished Rice, *Jing Mi*), 100g

Method of preparation & administration: Decoct the first 4 ingredients in water, remove the dregs, and reserve the liquid. Use this liquid to cook the rice into porridge and eat 2 times per day.

Added Flavors Three Immortals Congee
(*Jia Wei San Xian Zhou*)

Functions: Disperses accumulations and promotes digestion

Indications: Epigastric pain due to food stagnation and accumulation

Ingredients: Massa Medica Fermentata (*Shen Qu*), 12g, Fructus Crataegi (*Shan Zha*), 12g, Fructus Germinatus Hordei Vulgaris (*Mai Ya*), 12g, Fructus Germinatus Oryzae Sativae (*Gu Ya*), 12g, Pericarpium Citri Reticulatae (*Chen Pi*), 6g, Semen Oryzae Sativae (*i.e.*, Polished Rice, *Jing Mi*), 100g

Method of preparation & administration: Decoct the first 5 ingredients in water, remove the dregs, and reserve the liquid. Then cook the rice in this liquid into porridge and eat 2 times per day.

Evodia Congee
(*Wu Zhu Yu Zhou*)

Functions: Warms the center and stops pain, downbears counterflow and stops vomiting

Indications: Epigastric and abdominal chilly pain, *shan* pain, foot qi aching and pain, headache, vacuity cold enduring diarrhea

Ingredients: Fructus Evodiae Rutecarpae (*Wu Zhu Yu*), 3g, Semen

Oryzae Sativae (*i.e.*, Polished Rice, *Da Mi*), 50g, fresh Rhizoma Zingiberis (*i.e.*, Fresh Ginger, *Sheng Jiang*), 2 slices, Red Sugar (*i.e.*, Brown Sugar, *Hong Tang*), a suitable amount

Method of preparation & administration: First cook the rice into porridge. When half cooked, add the finely powdered Evodia and cook some more. Toward the end, add the fresh ginger and sugar to taste. Eat warm.

Sichuan Pepper Congee
(*Hua Jiao Zhou*)

Functions: Warms the center and nourishes the stomach, scatters cold and stops pain, kills worms (*i.e.*, parasites) and expels round-worms

Indications: Middle burner vacuity cold, epigastric and abdominal chilly pain, cold damp diarrhea, vomiting, *shan* pain, cold dysentery, roundworm disease

Ingredients: Powdered Fructus Zanthoxyli Bungeani (*Hua Jiao Fen*), 5g, Semen Oryzae Sativae (*i.e.*, Polished Rice, *Da Mi*), 50g, Granulated Sugar (*Sha Tang*), a suitable amount, Bulbus Allii Fistulosi (*i.e.*, Scallion, *Cong Bai*), 3 bulbs

Method of preparation & administration: First cook the rice into porridge as usual. Then add the sugar, scallions, and Sichuan pepper powder. Cook for 5-6 minutes more. Eat warm 2 times per day in the morning and evening.

Sichuan Pepper & Wheat Flour Congee
(*Jiao Mian Zhou*)

Functions: Warms the center and scatters cold, supplements the center and relaxes the stomach

Indications: Spleen/stomach vacuity cold, epigastric and abdominal chilly pain, stomach cold hiccup or vomiting, cold damp borborygmus and diarrhea

Ingredients: Fructus Zanthoxyli Bungeani (*Shu Jiao*), 5g, Wheat Flour (*Bai Mian Fen*), 150g, fresh Rhizoma Zingiberis (*i.e.*, Fresh Ginger, *Sheng Jiang*), 3 slices

Method of preparation & administration: Grind the Sichuan pepper into powder and cook it and the wheat flour into porridge. Add the ginger towards the end and cook for a few minutes more. Eat warm 1 time each morning and evening.

Contraindications: Because Sichuan pepper is greatly hot, do not eat this congee for prolonged periods of time. As soon as one is healed, stop.

Cabbage Congee
(*Yang Bai Cai Zhou*)

Functions: Relaxes cramping and stops pain

Indications: Cramping, aching, and pain of the stomach and abdomen

Ingredients: Chinese Cabbage (*Yang Bai Cai*), 500g, Semen Oryzae Sativae (*i.e.*, Polished Rice, *Jing Mi*), 50g

Method of preparation & administration: Wash the cabbage and cut it up into small pieces. Then cook it for 1/2 hour. Remove the cabbage and do not use it. Instead, cook the rice into porridge using the water left over from cooking the cabbage. Take 2 times per day.

Ume (*i.e.*, Preserved Salted Plum) Congee
(*Wu Mei Zhou*)

Functions: Boosts the qi and nourishes the stomach, engenders fluids and opens the stomach, quiets roundworms and expels worms (*i.e.*, parasites)

Indications: Stomach and epigastric cramping pain, dry mouth, devitalized appetite, red tongue with a scant coating, enduring diarrhea, enduring dysentery, hemafecia, hematuria, vexatious thirst, chronic gastritis, chronic colitis, intestinal roundworms

Ingredients: Fructus Pruni Mume (*Wu Mei*), 20g, Semen Oryzae Sativae (*i.e.*, Polished Rice, *Jing Mi*), 100g, Fructus Zizyphi Jujubae (*Hong Zao*), 3 pieces, Granulated Sugar (*Bing Tang*), a suitable amount

Method of preparation & administration: First decoct the preserved salted plum in 200ml of water down to 100ml. Remove the dregs and reserve the liquid. Add this to the rice, jujube, and sugar plus 600ml more water and cook into porridge. Eat warm each morning and evening.

Lily Bulb Congee
(*Bai He Zhou*)

Functions: Fortifies the spleen, nourishes the stomach, quiets the spirit

Indications: Stomach pain, pain under the heart, vexation and agitation, insomnia

Ingredients: Bulbus Lilii (*Bai He*), 60g, Semen Oryzae Sativae (*i.e.*, Polished Rice, *Jing Mi*), 100g, Red Sugar (*i.e.*, Brown Sugar, *Hong Tang*), a small amount

Method of preparation & administration: Cook the first two ingredients into porridge, add the brown sugar, and eat 1 time each day for 10 days.

12
Stomach & Duodenal Ulcers
(*Wei Ji Shi Er Zhi Chang Kui Yang*)

Polished Rice & Jujube Congee
(*Jing Mi Zao Zhou*)

Functions: Treats stomach and duodenal ulcers

Indications: Stomach and duodenal ulcers, acute gastritis. When used as a complement to other treatment its effect is good.

Ingredients: Semen Oryzae Sativae (*i.e.*, Polished Rice, *Jing Mi*), 100g, Fructus Zizyphi Jujubae (*Hong Zao*), 8 pieces

Method of preparation & administration: Cook into porridge as usual until it is very loose. Take every day.

13
Upper Digestive Tract Bleeding
(*Shang Xiao Hua Dao Chu Xue*)

Added Flavors Gardenia Fruit Congee
(*Jia Wei Zhi Zi Ren Zhou*)

Functions: Clears the liver, cools the blood, and stops bleeding

Indications: Liver fire upper digestive tract bleeding

Ingredients: Rhizoma Imperatae Cylindricae (*Bai Mao Gen*), 30g, fresh Rhizoma Nelumbinis Nuciferae (*Xian Ou*), 60g, powdered Fructus Gardeniae Jasminoidis (*Zhi Zi Ren Fen*), 6g, Semen Oryzae Sativae (*i.e.*, Polished Rice, *Jing Mi*), 100g

Method of preparation & administration: First decoct the Imperata in water, remove the dregs, and reserve the liquid. Then cook the rice and sliced, fresh lotus root into porridge using this liquid. When almost done, add the powdered Gardenia and cook a few minutes more. Eat 2 times per day.

Bletilla Congee
(Bai Ji Zhou)

Functions: Stops bleeding, disperses swelling, and engenders flesh

Indications: Lung and stomach bleeding disorders, pulmonary tuberculosis, stomach and duodenal ulcers

Ingredients: Powdered Rhizoma Bletillae Striatae (*Bai Ji Fen*), 15g, Semen Oryzae Glutinosae (*i.e.*, Glutinous Rice, *Nuo Mi*), 100g, Fructus Ziziphi Jujubae (*Da Zao*), 5 pieces, Honey (*Mi Tang*), 25g

Method of preparation & administration: Cook all these ingredients into porridge in 800ml of water. Eat warm 2 times per day. Ten days equal 1 course of treatment.

14
Thyroid Hypertrophy, Lymphadenopathy
(Jia Zhuang Xian Zhong Da, Lin Ba Jie He)

Mung Bean & Kelp Congee
(Lu Dou Hai Dai Zhou)

Functions: Clears, cools, and resolves toxins, disperses swelling and softens the hard

Indications: Concretions and conglomerations, thyroid hyperactivity during puberty, benign thyroid hypertrophy

Ingredients: Semen Phaseoli Mungonis (*i.e.*, Mung Beans, *Lu Dou*), 60g, Thallus Laminariae (*i.e.*, Kelp, *Hai Dai*), 30g, Semen Oryzae Sativae (*i.e.*, Polished Rice, *Da Mi*), 30g, Pericarpium Citri Reticulatae (*Chen Pi*), 6g, Red Sugar (*i.e.*, Brown Sugar, *Hong Tang*), 60g

Method of preparation & administration: First wash and soak till soft the kelp. Then put it in fresh water with the rice, mung beans, and orange peel and cook into porridge. Finally, add the brown sugar and eat.

15
Diabetes Mellitus (*Tang Niao Bing*)

Spinach Stalk Congee
(*Bo Cai Gen Zhou*)

Functions: Stops thirst, moistens dryness, nourishes the stomach

Indications: Diabetes mellitus

Ingredients: Spinach Stalk (*Bo Cai Gen*), 250g, Endothelium Corneum Gigeriae Galli (*Ji Nei Jin*), 10g, Semen Oryzae Sativae (*i.e.*, Polished Rice, *Da Mi*), 50g

Method of preparation & administration: Wash the spinach and cut into pieces. Add water and cook this and the Endothelium Corneum Gigeriae Galli for 30-40 minutes. Then add the rice and make into mushy porridge. Divide this into two doses and take both each day.

Radish Congee
(*Luo Bo Zhou*)

Functions: Rectifies the qi, transforms phlegm, clears heat, and disperses food

Indications: Wasting and thirsting, dry mouth, polyuria, obesity

Ingredients: Daikon Radish (*Luo Bo*), 5 whole ones, Semen Oryzae Sativae (*i.e.*, Polished Rice, *Jing Mi*), 250g

Method of preparation & administration: Cut up the radishes and boil in water. When soft, press out the juice and cook the rice in the resulting hot liquid. Cook into porridge and eat.

Hoovenia Fruit Congee
(*Zhi Ju Zi Zhou*)

Functions: Clears heat and eliminates vexation

Indications: Vexatious heat and oral thirst in the aftermath of febrile disease, inhibition of defecation and urination, vomiting due to alcohol intoxication

Ingredients: Fructus Hooveniae Dulcis (*Zhi Ju Zi*), 30g, Semen Oryzae Sativae (*i.e.*, Polished Rice, *Jing Mi*), 100g

Method of preparation & administration: First decoct the Fructus Hooveniae Dulcis, remove the dregs, and reserve the liquid. Then cook the rice in this liquid into porridge. Take on an empty stomach.

Rehmannia Congee
(*Di Huang Zhou*)

Functions: Enriches the liver and boosts the heart, clears heat and quiets the spirit

Indications: Damage to yin fluids in the aftermath of a febrile disease, vexatious heat and thirst, heat in the center of the hands, flushed cheeks in the evening, a dry mouth and desire for drinks, dry stools, insomnia

Ingredients: Fresh Radix Rehmanniae (*Xian Di Huang*), 50g (it is also ok to use *Sheng Di Huang*), Semen Zizyphi Spinosae (*Suan Zao Ren*), 30g, Semen Oryzae Sativae (*i.e.*, Polished Rice, *Jing Mi*), 100g

Method of preparation & administration: First decoct the Rehmannia and Zizyphus Spinosa in water, remove the dregs, and reserve the liquid. Then cook the rice in this liquid into porridge. Eat as one pleases.

Watermelon Seed Congee
(*Xi Gua Zi Zhou*)

Functions: Clears heat and nourishes the stomach, engenders fluids and stops thirst

Indications: Vexatious thirst and desire for drinks in the aftermath of a febrile disease

Ingredients: Semen Citrulli Vulgaris (*i.e.*, Watermelon Seed, *Xi Gua Zi*), 50g, Semen Oryzae Sativae (*i.e.*, Polished Rice, *Jing Mi*), 30g

Method of preparation & administration: Decoct the watermelon seeds in water, remove the dregs, and reserve the liquid. Then cook the rice in this liquid into porridge. Take as one pleases.

Sea Cucumber Congee
(*Hai Shen Zhou*)

Functions: Supplements the qi and nourishes yin, engender fluids and stops thirst

Indications: Qi and yin vacuity diabetes mellitus

Ingredients: Sea Cucumber (*Hai Shen*), 20g, Semen Oryzae Sativae (*i.e.*, Polished Rice, *Jing Mi*), 50g

Method of preparation & administration: Make into porridge as usual and eat.

Asparagus Congee
(*Tian Men Dong Zhou*)

Functions: Supplements the kidneys and enriches yin, nourishes the stomach and engenders fluids

Indications: Qi and yin vacuity diabetes mellitus

Ingredients: Tuber Asparagi Cochinensis (*Tian Men Dong*), 30g, Semen Oryzae Sativae (*i.e.*, Polished Rice, *Jing Mi*), 50g

Method of preparation & administration: Cook into porridge as usual and eat.

Chinese Yam & Longan Congee
(*Shan Yao Gui Yuan Zhou*)

Functions: Supplements the lungs, spleen, and kidneys

Indications: Upper, middle, and lower wasting and thirsting

Ingredients: Radix Dioscoreae Oppositae (*Shan Yao*), Arillus Euphoriae Longanae (*Long Yan Rou*), Fructus Litchi Sinensis (*Li Zhi*), Fructus Schizandrae Chinensis (*Wu Wei Zi*), suitable amounts of each

Method of preparation & administration: Make into porridge as usual.

16
Anemia (*Pin Xue*)

Lamb Shinbone Congee
(*Yang Jing Gu Zhou*)

Functions: Supplements vacuity detriment

Indications: Anemia

Ingredients: Lamb Shinbone (*Yang Jing Gu*), 2 pieces, Fructus Zizyphi Jujubae (*Hong Zao*), 20 pieces, Semen Oryzae Sativae (*i.e.*, Polished Rice, *Jing Mi*), 100g

Method of preparation & administration: Break open the lamb bone to expose the marrow. Add water, the jujubes, and rice and cook into porridge. Divide into 2 portions and take each day. One half month equals 1 course of treatment.

Jujube Congee
(*Da Zao Zhou*)

Functions: Fortifies the spleen and boosts the qi

Indications: Spleen and stomach vacuity weakness, anemia, stomach vacuity lack of appetite, etc.

Ingredients: Fructus Zizyphi Jujubae (*Da Zao*), 10 pieces, Semen Oryzae Sativae (*i.e.*, Polished Rice, *Jing Mi*), 100g, Crystallized Sugar (*Bing Tang*), a suitable amount

Method of preparation & administration: Cook the rice and jujubes together in water to make a porridge and then add sugar to taste. Eat warm.

Immortal Human Congee
(*Xian Ren Zhou*)

Functions: Supplements the liver and kidneys and nourishes the blood

Indications: Liver blood/kidney yin vacuity anemia

Ingredients: Radix Polygoni Multiflori (*He Shou Wu*), 60g, Semen Oryzae Sativae (*i.e.*, Polished Rice, *Jing Mi*), 60g, Fructus Zizyphi Jujubae (*Da Zao*), 3-5 pieces, Red Sugar (*i.e.*, Brown Sugar, *Hong Tang*), a suitable amount

Method of preparation & administration: First decoct the Polygonum, remove the dregs, and reserve the liquid. Then use this liquid plus additional water to make porridge from the rice and jujubes. Add the sugar at the end and bring to a boil 1 or 2 more times.

Glutinous Rice & Donkey Skin Glue Congee (*Nuo Mi E Jiao Zhou*)

Functions: Supplement the spleen and heart, nourishes the blood

Indications: Spleen and heart dual vacuity anemia

Ingredients: Gelatinum Corii Asini (*E Jiao*), 30g, Semen Oryzae Glutinosae (*i.e.*, Glutinous Rice, *Nuo Mi*), 60g, Red Sugar (*i.e.*, Brown Sugar, *Hong Tang*), a small amount

Method of preparation & administration: Make the rice into porridge as usual. Grind the donkey skin glue into a fine powder and add it and the sugar to the porridge when almost done. Mix thoroughly and bring to a boil 1-2 more times.

17
High Blood Pressure (*Gao Xue Ya Bing*)

Preserved Egg & Mussel Congee (*Song Hua Dan Cai Zhou*)

Functions: Clears the heart and downbears fire

Indications: High blood pressure, tinnitus, dizziness and vertigo, toothache

Ingredients: Preserved Egg (*Song Hua*), 1 whole one, (dry) Mussels (*Dan Cai*), 50g, Semen Oryzae Sativae (*i.e.*, Polished Rice, *Da Mi*), 50g

Method of preparation & administration: First remove the shell of the preserved egg and soak the (dry) mussels in water until soft. Then put the preserved egg and mussels together with rice and water and cook into porridge. One may add a small amount of salt to taste. Eat the mussels and drink the porridge each morning on an empty stomach.

Celery Congee
(Qin Cai Zhou)

Functions: Clears liver heat, downbears blood pressure

Indications: High blood pressure, dizziness, headache

Ingredients: Celery (*Qin Cai*), 120g, Semen Oryzae Sativae (*i.e.*, Polished Rice, *Jing Mi*), 250g, Salt (*Yan*), a suitable amount

Method of preparation & administration: Wash the celery and cut the stalks into pieces. Cook with the rice in water to make porridge. Salt to taste and eat regularly.

Chrysanthemum & Hawthorne Berry Congee
(Ju Hua Shan Zha Zhou)

Functions: Clears liver heat and downbears blood pressure

Indications: Liver yang hyperactivity high blood pressure, high cholesterol, coronary heart disease

Ingredients: Flos Chrysanthemi Morifolii (*Ju Hua*), 12g, Fructus Crataegi (*Shan Zha*), 12g, Semen Oryzae Sativae (*i.e.*, Polished Rice, *Jing Mi*), 60g, Granulated Sugar (*Bing Tang*), a suitable amount

Method of preparation & administration: Grind the first 2 ingredients into powder. Make porridge out of the rice, 500ml of water, and sugar. When the rice soup begins to boil but has not yet thickened, add the powdered ingredients. Cook over a slow fire for some time more. Eat warm, 1-2 times per day.

Contraindications: Do not take in winter.

Pork Brains & Gastrodia Congee
(Zhu Nao Tian Ma Zhou)

Functions: Dispels head wind, supplements the brain marrow, settles tremor, settles pain

Indications: High blood pressure, arteriosclerosis, liver wind internally stirring

Ingredients: Pork Brains (Zhu Nao), 1 whole one, Rhizoma Gastrodiae Elatae (Tian Ma), 10g, Semen Oryzae Sativae (i.e. Polished Rice, Jing Mi), 250g

Method of preparation & administration: Grind the Gastrodia into a fine powder and cook with the rice and water into porridge. Add the pork brains and cook till done. Eat warm 1 time per day.

18
High Cholesterol (Gao Zhi Xue Zheng)

Alisma Congee
(Ze Xie Zhou)

Functions: Reduces blood fat

Indications: Hyperlipidemia

Ingredients: Powdered Rhizoma Alismatis (Ze Xie Fen), 10g, Semen Oryzae Sativae (i.e., Polished Rice, Jing Mi), 50g

Method of preparation & administration: Cook the rice into porridge in 500ml of water. Add the powdered Alisma and mix thoroughly. Bring to a boil several times more and eat warm 2 times per day.

Polygonum Multiflorum Congee
(He Shou Wu Zhou)

Functions: Reduces blood fat

Indications: Hyperlipidemia

Ingredients: Powdered Radix Polygoni Multiflori (*He Shou Wu Fen*), 30g, Fructus Zizyphi Jujubae (*Da Zao*), 2 pieces, Semen Oryzae Sativae (*i.e.*, Polished Rice, *Jing Mi*), 50g, White Sugar (*Bai Tang*), a suitable amount

Method of preparation & administration: Cook the rice and jujubes into porridge in 500ml of water. Then mix in the Polygonum powder and bring to a boil several times again. Finally, add some sugar to taste and eat warm, 2 times per day, morning and evening.

Mussel Congee
(Dan Cai Zhou)

Functions: Reduces blood fat and blood pressure

Indications: Hyperlipidemia and high blood pressure

Ingredients: Dry Mussels (*Gan Dan Cai*), 50g, Semen Oryzae Sativae (*i.e.*, Polished Rice, *Jing Mi*), 100g

Method of preparation & administration: Soak the dry mussels in water for 1/2 day. Boil them a bit and remove their hearts. Add to the rice and 800ml of water and cook into porridge. Add a small amount of cooking oil and salt and eat warm, 2 times per day, morning and evening. Eat regularly over a long period of time.

Five Flours Congee
(Wu Mi Fen Zhou)

Functions: Boosts the lungs and quiets the heart, rectifies the center and opens the stomach

Indications: Hyperlipidemia, coronary heart disease, arteriosclerosis, and the prevention of cancer

Ingredients: Powdered Semen Zeae Maydis (*i.e.*, Corn Flour, *Wu Mi Fen*), Semen Oryzae Sativae (*i.e.*, Polished Rice, *Jing Mi*), suitable amounts each

Method of preparation & administration: Mix a suitable amount of corn flour in cold water and add to rice porridge. Bring to a boil again and eat warm for breakfast or supper.

19
Coronary Heart Disease (*Guan Xin Bing*)

Allium Bulb & Hawthorne Berry Congee
(*Xie Bai Shan Zha Zhou*)

Functions: Frees the flow of yang and disperses cold phlegm, moves the qi and quickens the blood, downbears the qi and stops pain

Indications: Coronary heart disease with chest pain and angina pectoris

Ingredients: Bulbus Allii Macrostemi (*Xie Bai*), 9g, Fructus Crataegi (*Shan Zha*), 12g, Semen Oryzae Sativae (*i.e.*, Polished Rice, *Jing Mi*), 100g

Method of preparation & administration: Make into porridge as usual. Eat 1-2 times per day.

Garlic Congee
(*Da Suan Zhou*)

Functions: Scatters cold and dispels stasis, moves the qi and stops pain

Indications: Hyperlipidemia with chest pain due to coronary artery disease accompanied by cold symptoms

Ingredients: Garlic (*Da Suan*), 30g, Semen Oryzae Sativae (*i.e.*, Polished Rice, *Jing Mi*), 100g

Method of preparation & administration: Put the garlic in boiling water for 1 minute to blanch, and peel. Then put the rice in the same boiling water and cook into porridge. Put the garlic back in the porridge, continue cooking, mix well, and make into gruel. Take warm each morning and evening.

Polygonum Multiflorum & Lily Bulb Congee (*Shou Wu Bai He Zhou*)

Functions: Enriches yin and supplements the heart

Indications: Coronary heart disease in those with yin vacuity

Ingredients: Radix Polygoni Multiflori (*He Shou Wu*), 30g, Bulbus Lilii (*Bai He*), 30g, Fructus Lycii Chinensis (*Gou Qi Zi*), 9g, Fructus Zizyphi Jujubae (*Da Zao*), 6 pieces, Semen Oryzae Sativae (*i.e.*, Polished Rice, *Jing Mi*), 100g

Method of preparation & administration: First decoct the Polygonum Multiflorum in water, remove the dregs, and reserve the liquid. Then cook all the rest of the ingredients in this liquid into porridge. Take in the morning and evening.

Ginger, Cinnamon & Allium Bulb Congee (*Jiang Gui Xie Bai Zhou*)

Functions: Scatters cold and moves the qi, quickens the blood and stops pain

Indications: Coronary heart disease with chest pain and angina pectoris

Ingredients: Dry Rhizoma Zingiberis (*Gan Jiang*), 3g, Bulbus Allii (*Xie Bai*), 9g, Bulbus Allii Fistulosi (*i.e.*, Scallion, *Cong Bai*), 2 bulbs, Semen Oryzae Sativae (*i.e.*, Polished Rice, *Jing Mi*), 100, powdered Cortex Cinnamomi (*Rou Gui Fen*), 1g

Method of preparation & administration: Make the first 4 ingredients into porridge. When the porridge is cooked, sprinkle the cinnamon powder over the top and eat 1-2 times per day.

20
Congestive Heart Failure
(*Chong Xue Xing Xin Li Shuai Jie*)

Longan & Lily Bulb Congee
(*Yuan Rou Bai He Zhou*)

Functions: Supplements the heart, nourishes the blood, and enriches yin

Indications: Heart qi, blood, and yin vacuity with frequent palpitations and shortness of breath

Ingredients: Arillus Euphoriae Longanae (*Long Yan Rou*), 15g, Bulbus Lilii (*Bai He*), 15g, Fructus Zizyphi Jujubae (*Da Zao*), 6 pieces, Semen Oryzae Sativae (*i.e.*, Polished Rice, *Jing Mi*), 100g, White Sugar (*Bai Tang*), a suitable amount

Method of preparation & administration: Make into porridge as usual and take 2 times per day in the morning and evening.

Lotus Seed & Zizyphus Spinosa Congee
(*Lian Zi Suan Zao Zhou*)

Functions: Supplements the heart, spleen, liver, and kidneys and clears heat

Indications: Heart qi, blood, and yin vacuity with vacuity heat

Ingredients: Semen Nelumbinis Nuciferae (*Lian Zi*, without the center), 30g, Semen Zizyphi Spinosae (*Suan Zao Ren*), 30g, Fructus Zizyphi Jujubae (*Da Zao*), 6 pieces, Semen Oryzae Sativae (*i.e.*,

Polished Rice, *Jing Mi*), 100g, White Sugar (*Bai Tang*), a suitable amount

Method of preparation & administration: Make into porridge as usual and eat 2 times per day in the morning and evening.

Cinnamon, Ginger & Ginseng Congee (*Gui Jiang Ren Shen Zhou*)

Functions: Supplements heart qi and warms yang

Indications: Heart yang vacuity with palpitations, shortness of breath, fatigued spirit, exhaustion, lack of warmth in the four limbs

Ingredients: Ramulus Cinnamomi (*Gui Zhi*), 6g, dry Rhizoma Zingiberis (*Gan Jiang*), 6g, Radix Panacis Ginseng (*Ren Shen*), 3g, Fructus Zizyphi Jujubae (*Da Zao*), 8 pieces, Semen Oryzae Sativae (*i.e.*, Polished Rice, *Jing Mi*), 100g, Red Sugar (*i.e.*, Brown Sugar, *Hong Tang*), a suitable amount

Method of preparation & administration: Decoct the first 4 ingredients, remove the dregs, and reserve the liquid. Then make porridge with the rice and this liquid. Add the brown sugar when cooked and eat 2 times per day in the morning and evening.

Ginseng, Astragalus & Aconite Congee (*Shen Qi Fu Zi Zhou*)

Functions: Supplements heart qi and warms yang

Indications: Heart yang vacuity with palpitations, shortness of the breath, fatigue and exhaustion

Ingredients: Radix Praeparatus Aconiti Carmichaeli (*Zhi Fu Zi*), 6g, Radix Panacis Ginseng (*Ren Shen*), 3g, Radix Astragali Membranacei (*Huang Qi*), 15g, Fructus Zizyphi Jujubae (*Da Zao*), 8 pieces, Semen

Oryzae Sativae (*i.e.*, Polished Rice, *Jing Mi*), 100g, Red Sugar (*i.e.*, Brown Sugar, *Hong Tang*), a suitable amount

Method of preparation & administration: First decoct the Aconite for 1 1/2-2 hours. Then put in the Ginseng, Astragalus, and jujube. Decoct these for another 40 minutes, remove the dregs, and reserve the liquid. Make porridge with this liquid and the rice and add the brown sugar at the end to taste. Take 2 times per day in the morning and evening.

Fragrant Solomon's Seal Congee (*Yu Zhu Zhou*)

Functions: Nourishes yin and moistens dryness

Indications: Congestive heart failure due to rheumatic heart disease, congestive heart disease or pulmonary heart disease characterized as lung and stomach yin vacuity with cough, dry throat, irritability, and thirst

Ingredients: Rhizoma Polygonati Odorati (*Yu Zhu*), 15g, Semen Oryzae Sativae (*i.e.*, Polished Rice, *Jing Mi*), 100g, Granulated Sugar (*Bing Tang*), a small amount

Method of preparation & administration: First decoct the Fragrant Solomon's Seal, remove the dregs, and reserve the liquid. Then make porridge with the rice and this liquid. Add the sugar at the end of cooking and eat 2 times per day in the morning and evening. Five to 7 days equal 1 course of treatment.

21
Chronic Low Blood Pressure
(*Man Xing Di Xue Ya*)

Added Flavors Engender the Pulse Congee (*Jia Wei Sheng Mai Zhou*)

Functions: Fortifies the spleen and boosts the qi

Indications: Chronic low blood pressure due to qi and yin vacuity

Ingredients: Radix Panacis Ginseng (*Ren Shen*), 6g, Tuber O-phiopogonis Japonicae (*Mai Men Dong*), 15g, Rhizoma Polygonati (*Huang Jing*), 15g, Pericarpium Citri Reticulatae (*Chen Pi*), 12g, mix-fried Radix Glycyrrhizae (*Zhi Gan Cao*), 9g, Fructus Schizandrae Chinensis (*Wu Wei Zi*), 6g, Semen Oryzae Sativae (*i.e.*, Polished Rice, *Jing Mi*), 100g

Method of preparation & administration: First decoct in water all the ingredients except the rice. Remove the dregs and reserve the liquid. Use the resulting liquid to make the rice into porridge. Eat 2 times per day.

22
Wind Stroke Disease (*Zhong Feng Bing*)

Cannabis Seed Congee
(*Dong Ma Zi Zhou*)

Functions: Dispels wind, moistens the intestines

Indications: Hemiplegia due to wind stoke, aphasia, paralysis of the hands and feet, constipation

Ingredients: Semen Cannabis Sativae (*Dong Ma Zi*), 30g, Spica Seu Flos Schizonepetae Tenuifoliae (*Jing Jie Sui*), Herba Menthae (*Bo He Ye*), 6g, Semen Setariae Italicae (*i.e.*, Millet, *Bai Su Mi*), 100g

Method of preparation & administration: First decoct the Schi-zonepeta and Mentha and reserve the liquid. Then cook the Cannabis seeds and millet in this liquid into porridge. Eat on an empty stomach.

Lamb Tripe & Rice Congee
(*Yang Du Jing Mi Zhou*)

Functions: Enriches and supplements the spleen and stomach

Indications: Bodily vacuity weakness after a wind stroke

Ingredients: Lamb Tripe (*Yang Du*), 1 whole one, Semen Oryzae Sativae (*i.e.*, Polished Rice, *Jing Mi*), 250g, Fructus Zanthoxyli Bungeani (*i.e.*, Sichuan Pepper, *Hua Jiao*), Semen Praeparatum Sojae (*i.e.*, Fermented Soybeans, *Dou Chi*), Bulbus Allii Fistulosi (*i.e.*, Scallion, *Cong*), and Rhizoma Zingiberis (*i.e.*, Ginger, *Jiang*), a small amount each

Method of preparation & administration: Make into porridge as usual. Each day take 2 times.

Schizonepeta & Millet Congee
(*Jing Jie Su Mi Zhou*)

Functions: Quickens the blood, dispels wind

Indications: Wind stroke, aphasia and indistinct speech, clouded consciousness, eyes and mouth awry

Ingredients: Spica Seu Flos Schizonepetae Tenuifoliae (*Jing Jie Sui*), 15g, Herba Menthae (*Bo He Ye*), 15g, Semen Praeparatum Sojae (*i.e.*, Fermented Soybean, *Dou Chi*), 50g, Semen Setariae Italicae (*i.e.*, Millet, *Bai Su Mi*), 100g

Method of preparation & administration: First decoct the first 3 ingredients, remove the dregs, and reserve the liquid. Then add the millet and cook into porridge. Take on an empty stomach each day.

23
Neurasthenia (*Shen Jing Shuai Ruo*)

Rice & Coix Congee
(*Jing Mi Yi Ren Zhou*)

Functions: Supplements the center, boosts the qi, quiets the heart

Indications: Spirit channel deficiency weakness conditions

Ingredients: Semen Oryzae Sativae (*i.e.*, Polished Rice, *Jing Mi*), 100g, Semen Coicis Lachryma-jobi (*Yi Mi Ren*), 50g, Fructus Zizyphi Jujubae (*Hong Zao*), 10 pieces

Method of preparation & administration: Make into porridge as usual. Take 1 time each day.

Poria Congee
(*Fu Ling Zhou*)

Functions: Tranquilizes the heart and quiets the spirit

Indications: Insomnia; patient wants to go to sleep but cannot get to sleep

Ingredients: Sclerotium Poriae Cocos (*Fu Ling*), 50g, Semen Oryzae Sativae (*i.e.*, Polished Rice, *Jing Mi*), 100g

Method of preparation & administration: First cook the rice into porridge. Then powder the Poria and add. Cook some more and eat.

Zizyphus Spinosa Congee
(*Suan Zao Ren Zhou*)

Functions: Nourishes yin, supplements the heart, and quiets the spirit

Indications: Heart palpitations, insomnia, excessive dreams due to heart/spleen dual vacuity

Ingredients: Semen Zizyphi Spinosae (*Suan Zao Ren*), 15g, Semen Oryzae Sativae (*i.e.*, Polished Rice, *Jing Mi*), 100g

Method of preparation & administration: Stir-fry the Zizyphus Spinosa until yellow and then grind into powder. Cook the rice into porridge. While still hot, add the powdered Zizyphus Spinosa, cook some more, and eat on an empty stomach.

Biota Seed Congee
(*Bai Zi Ren Zhou*)

Functions: Enriches, nourishes, and strengthens the body, nourishes the heart and moistens the intestines

Indications: Palpitations, insomnia, constipation, poor memory, bodily weakness, dry intestines constipation

Ingredients: Semen Biotae Orientalis (*Bai Zi Ren*), 15g, Semen Oryzae Sativae (*i.e.*, Polished Rice, *Jing Mi*), 60g, Honey (*Mi Tang*), a suitable amount

Method of preparation & administration: Pound the Biota seeds to crack them open and make into porridge with the rice. Add honey when the porridge is almost done and continue cooking a few minutes more. Eat 2 times per day in the morning and evening. Two to 3 days equal 1 course of treatment.

Note: Substitute Semen Juglandis Regiae (*i.e.*, Walnut, *Hu Tao Ren*) for honey in the weak and elderly.

Contraindications: This congee should not be eaten by those with loose stools or fever.

Dragon Bone Congee
(*Long Gu Zhou*)

Functions: Settles fright and represses yang, astringes and secures

Indications: Heart spirit not quiet, heart palpitations, insomnia, spermatorrhea, postpartum vacuity sweating which will not stop, night sweats, spontaneous sweating, profuse uterine bleeding, etc.

Ingredients: Quartz (*i.e.*, Rock Crystal, *Bai Shi Ying*), 10g, Semen Oryzae Glutinosae (*i.e.*, Glutinous Rice, *Nuo Mi*), 50g

Method of preparation & administration: First powder the crystal and wash in water till clear. Decoct in water, remove the dregs, and reserve the liquid. Add to the rice and more water and cook into porridge as usual. Take warm morning and evening on an empty stomach.

Wheat Congee
(*Xiao Mai Zhou*)

Functions: Nourishes heart qi, stops vacuity sweating, boosts the liver and stops thirst

Indications: Heart qi insufficiency with palpitations, shortness of breath, spontaneous sweating, oral thirst, lack of strength, fatigue, etc.

Ingredients: Fructus Tritici (*i.e.*, Wheat, *Xiao Mai*), 50g

Method of preparation & administration: Cook into porridge as usual and eat.

Note: Fresh wheat is categorized as warm, while aged wheat is categorized as cool. Therefore, in summer it is appropriate to eat aged wheat, but after the fall it is appropriate to eat fresh wheat.

Albizzia Flower Congee
(He Huan Hua Zhou)

Functions: Nourishes heart blood and quiets the spirit, opens the channels and network vessels

Indications: Insomnia, emotional depression, vacuity vexation, restlessness, poor memory, detriment and damage due to fall and strike, bone break, swelling, and pain

Ingredients: Dry Flos Albizziae Julibrissinis (Gan He Huan Hua), 30g, Semen Oryzae Sativae (i.e., Polished Rice, Jing Mi), 50g, Red Sugar (i.e., Brown Sugar, Hong Tang), a suitable amount

Method of preparation & administration: Make the rice in porridge as usual, stir in the Albizzia flowers, and add sugar to taste. Eat warm on an empty stomach each evening 1 hour before going to bed.

Caulis Polygoni Multiflori Congee
(Ye Jiao Teng Zhou)

Functions: Nourishes the blood and quiets the spirit, dispels wind and opens the network vessels

Indications: Vacuity vexation, insomnia, habitual insomnia, excessive dreams, wind damp bi pain

Ingredients: Caulis Polygoni Multiflori (Ye Jiao Teng), 60g, Fructus Zizyphi Jujubae (Da Zao), 2 pieces, Semen Oryzae Sativae (i.e., Polished Rice, Jing Mi), 50g, White Sugar (Bai Tang), a suitable amount

Method of preparation & administration: First decoct the Caulis Polygoni Multiflori in 500ml of water, remove the dregs, and reserve the liquid. Add the rice, sugar, and jujubes and another 200ml of hot water and cook into porridge. Eat warm 1 hour before bed each evening.

Codonopsis & Fragrant Solomon's Seal Congee
(Dang Shen Yu Zhu Zhou)

Functions: Supplements and nourishes heart qi and yin

Indications: Qi and yin insufficiency heart disease, fatigue, lack of strength, spontaneous sweating, heart palpitations, dry mouth, heat in the centers of the hands and feet, night sweats, insomnia, excessive dreams, red cheeks or lips, a red tongue and a fine, rapid pulse

Ingredients: Radix Codonopsis Pilosulae (*Dang Shen*), 30g, Rhizoma Polygonati Odorati (*Yu Zhu*), 20g, Semen Oryzae Sativae (*i.e.*, Polished Rice, *Da Mi*), 50g

Method of preparation & administration: Decoct the first 2 ingredients in water, remove the dregs, and reserve the liquid. Add water and the rice and cook into porridge as usual. Eat warm 2 times per day.

Contraindications: Common cold, water swelling, abdominal distention, torpid appetite

24
Acute & Chronic Hepatitis, Liver & Spleen Hypertrophy
(Ji Man Xing Gan Yan, Gan Pi Zhong Da)

Perilla Seed & Rice Congee
(Zi Su Da Mi Zhou)

Functions: Clears heat, dispels dampness

Indications: Icteric hepatitis

Ingredients: Fructus Perillae Frutescentis (*Zi Su Zi*), 1 kg, Semen Oryzae Sativae (*i.e.*, Polished Rice, *Da Mi*), 150g

Method of preparation & administration: First wash the Perilla seeds and grind. Then add to the rice and make into porridge. Begin by taking several times per day.

Artemisia Capillaris Congee (*Yin Chen Zhou*)

Functions: Clears heat and eliminates dampness

Indications: Acute icteric and infectious hepatitis

Ingredients: Herba Artemisiae Capillaris (*Yin Chen Hao*), 45g, Semen Oryzae Sativae (*i.e.*, Polished Rice, *Jing Mi*), 100g, White Sugar (*Bai Tang*), a small amount

Method of preparation & administration: Decoct the Artemisia Capillaris in 200ml of water down to 100ml. Remove the dregs and add the rice. Also add another 600ml of water and cook into porridge. Add a small amount of sugar and continue cooking for a few minutes more. Take 2-3 times per day. Seven to 10 days equal 1 course of treatment.

25
Cirrhosis (*Gan Bian Hua*)

Compound Peach Seed Congee (*Fu Fang Tao Ren Zhou*)

Functions: Quickens the blood and transforms stasis

Indications: Early cirrhosis due to qi and blood stagnation and stasis

Ingredients: Semen Pruni Persicae (*Tao Ren*), 9g, Pericarpium Citri Reticulatae (*Chen Pi*), 6g, Fructus Crataegi (*Shan Zha*), 12g, Semen Oryzae Sativae (*i.e.*, Polished Rice, *Jing Mi*), 100g

Method of preparation & administration: Decoct the first 3 ingredients in water, remove the dregs, and reserve the liquid. Cook the rice in this liquid into porridge and eat 2 times per day.

Citron, Buddha's Hand & Radish Seed Congee (*Xiang Fo Lai Fu Zhou*)

Functions: Moves the qi and disperses distention

Indications: Cirrhosis of the liver with tympanites due to qi stagnation

Ingredients: Fructus Citri (*Xiang Yuan*, a type of Citron), 9g, Fructus Citri Sacrodactylis (*Fo Shou*), 9g, powdered Semen Raphani Sativi (*Lai Fu Zi Fen*), 15g, Semen Oryzae Sativae (*i.e.*, Polished Rice, *Jing Mi*), 100g

Method of preparation & administration: Decoct the first 2 ingredients in water, remove the dregs, and reserve the liquid. Cook the rice and radish seed powder into porridge using this liquid. Eat 2 times per day.

Red Peony, Peach Seed, Cinnamon & Poria Congee (*Chi Tao Gui Ling Zhou*)

Functions: Quickens the blood and transforms stasis

Indications: Tympanites due to blood stasis accompanying cirrhosis

Ingredients: Radix Rubrus Paeoniae Lactiflorae (*Chi Shao*), 9g, Semen Pruni Persicae (*Tao Ren*), 9g, Radix Angelicae Sinensis (*Dang Gui*), 9g, Fructus Polygoni Orientalis (*Shui Hong Hua Zi*), 6g, Pericarpium Citri Reticulatae (*Chen Pi*), 6g, Sclerotium Poriae Cocos (*Fu Ling*), 12g, Sclerotium Polypori Umbellati (*Zhu Ling*), 12g, Semen Phaseoli Calcarati (*i.e.*, Aduki Beans, *Chi Xiao Dou*), 30g, Semen Oryzae Sativae (*i.e.*, Polished Rice, *Jing Mi*), 60g

Method of preparation & administration: Decoct the first 7 ingredients in water, remove the dregs, and reserve the liquid. Then cook the aduki beans and rice in this liquid into porridge and eat 2 times per day.

26
Superficial Edema, Ascites
(*Fu Zhong, Fu Shui*)

Black Bean Congee
(*Wu Dou Zhou*)

Functions: Expels wind and quickens the blood, disinhibits water and disperses swelling

Indications: Water swelling, distention, and fullness, wind damp *bi* pain, inhibition of the joints due to pain, swelling, toxic ulcers, etc.

Ingredients: Semen Glycinis Hispidae (*i.e.*, Black Soybeans, *Wu Dou*), 30g, Semen Oryzae Sativae (*i.e.*, Polished Rice, *Jing Mi*), 100g, Red Sugar (*i.e.*. Brown Sugar, *Hong Tang*), a suitable amount

Method of preparation & administration: Soak the black soybeans overnight in warm water. Then cook with the rice into porridge using 1,000ml of water. Add brown sugar to taste and eat each morning warm. Can be eaten for a long period of time.

Compound Aduki Bean Congee
(*Fu Fang Chi Dou Zhou*)

Functions: Disinhibits water and promotes urination

Indications: Ascites due to cirrhosis

Ingredients: Semen Phaseoli Calcarati (*i.e.* Aduki Beans, *Chi Xiao Dou*), 30g, Semen Coicis Lachryma-jobi (*Yi Yi Ren*), 30g, powdered

Pericarpium Citri Reticulatae (*Chen Pi*), 6g, Semen Oryzae Sativae (*i.e.*, Polished Rice, *Jing Mi*), 30g

Method of preparation & administration: Cook all the above ingredients into porridge as usual and eat 2 times per day.

Pork Liver & Mung Bean Congee (*Zhu Gan Lu Dou Zhou*)

Functions: Disinhibits water and disperses swelling

Indications: Superficial edema, inhibited urination, and other such conditions

Ingredients: Semen Phaseoli Mungonis (*i.e.*, Mung Beans, *Lu Dou*), 50g, Semen Oryzae Sativae (*i.e.*, Polished Rice, *Da Mi*), fresh Pork Liver (*Xian Zhu Gan*), 100g

Method of preparation & administration: First wash the rice and mung beans. Add a suitable amount of water and cook into porridge. Puree the pork liver and add to the porridge and cook a little longer. Do not add salt.

Imperata Cylindrica & Rice Congee (*Mao Gen Da Mi Zhou*)

Functions: Disinhibits water and disperses swelling

Indications: Water swelling, inhibited urination and other such conditions

Ingredients: Fresh Rhizoma Imperatae Cylindricae (*Xian Mao Gen*), 200g (if using dry, 50g), Semen Oryzae Sativae (*i.e.*, Polished Rice, *Da Mi*), 150g

Method of preparation & administration: First decoct the Imperata in a suitable amount of water. After the water has boiled 1/2 hour, remove the dregs. Then add the rice to this liquid and cook into porridge. Each day divide into 2 portions and eat both.

Areca Seed Congee
(*Bing Lang Zhou*)

Functions: Moves the qi, disinhibits water, and disperses swelling

Indications: Abdominal distention and oppression, bowel movements not crisp, possible foot qi, water swelling, etc.

Ingredients: Semen Arecae Catechu (*Bing Lang*), 10g, Semen Oryzae Sativae (*i.e.*, Polished Rice, *Jing Mi*), 100g, Honey (*Mi Tang*) or Ginger Juice (*Jiang Zhi*), a suitable amount

Method of preparation & administration: First decoct the Areca Catechu, remove the dregs, and reserve the liquid. Then cook the rice into porridge using this liquid. While still hot, stir in some ginger juice or honey. Eat on an empty stomach.

Duck Meat & Rice Congee
(*Ya Rou Da Mi Zhou*)

Functions: Enriches yin and supplements vacuity, disinhibits water and disperses swelling

Indications: Water swelling diseases

Ingredients: Male Duck Meat (*Xiong Ya Rou*), Semen Oryzae Sativae (*i.e.*, Polished Rice, *Da Mi*), suitable amounts

Method of preparation & administration: Cook these two ingredients together into porridge. Add a little salt to flavor. Eat 2 times each day.

Corn, Dolichos & Jujube Congee
(Yu Mi Dou Zao Zhou)

Functions: Nourishes and constructs

Indications: Unhealthy water swelling conditions

Ingredients: Semen Zeae Maydis (*i.e., Corn, Yu Mi*), 50g, Semen Dolichos Lablabis (*Bai Bian Dou*), 25g, Fructus Zizyphi Jujubae (*Da Zao*), 50g

Method of preparation & administration: Cook into porridge as usual. Take 1 time per day.

White Poria Congee
(Bai Fu Ling Zhou)

Functions: Fortifies the spleen and disinhibits dampness

Indications: Superficial edema in the elderly, obesity, inhibited urination, diarrhea, etc.

Ingredients: Sclerotium Poriae Cocos (*Bai Fu Ling*), 15g, Semen Oryzae Sativae (*i.e.*, Polished Rice, *Jing Mi*), 100g, Salt (*Yan*), a suitable amount, powdered Fructus Piperis Nigri (*i.e.*, Black Pepper, *Hu Jiao*), a suitable amount

Method of preparation & administration: First wash the rice and powder the Poria. Add together and cook into porridge with water. Then add salt and pepper to taste. Eat frequently.

Coix Congee
(Yi Mi Ren)

Functions: Fortifies the spleen and eliminates dampness

Indications: Spleen and stomach vacuity weakness, rheumatic arthritis, water swelling, warts, etc.

Ingredients: Semen Coicis Lachryma-jobi (*Yi Yi Mi*), 50g, White Sugar (*Bai Tang*), a suitable amount

Method of preparation & administration: Cook the Coix in a suitable amount of water to make porridge and then add some sugar and eat.

Aduki Bean Congee
(*Chi Xiao Dou Zhou*)

Functions: Fortifies the spleen and disinhibits water

Indications: Water swelling diseases, foot qi dampness, obesity

Ingredients: Semen Phaseoli Calcarati (*i.e.* Aduki Beans, *Chi Xiao Dou*), 50g, Semen Oryzae Sativae (*i.e.*, Polished Rice, *Jing Mi*), 200g, Salt (*Yan*), a suitable amount

Method of preparation & administration: Cook the rice and Aduki beans together in a suitable amount of water to make into porridge. Add salt to taste and eat regularly.

Alisma Congee
(*Ze Xie Zhou*)

Functions: Disinhibits water and percolates dampness, discharges heat

Indications: Water dampness stoppage and stagnation, inhibited urination, water swelling, lower burner damp heat vaginal discharge, urinary strangury and astringency, high blood pressure, high cholesterol, diabetes mellitus, and chronic liver disease

Ingredients: Powdered Rhizoma Alismatis (*Ze Xie Fen*), 10g, Semen Oryzae Sativae (*i.e.*, Polished Rice, *Jing Mi*), 50g

Method of preparation & administration: First cook the rice into porridge in 500ml of water. Stir in the Alisma powder and cook a while longer. Eat warm 2 times per day. Three days equal 1 course of treatment.

Morning Glory Seed Congee
(Qian Niu Zi Zhou)

Functions: Discharges water and disperses swelling, opens the stools and descends the qi

Indications: Water swelling and distention, abdominal water distention and fullness, inhibited urination, constipation, foot qi, superficial edema, etc.

Ingredients: Powdered Semen Pharbiditis (*Qian Niu Zi*), 1g, Semen Oryzae Sativae (*i.e.*, Polished Rice, *Da Mi*), 100g, fresh Rhizoma Zingiberis (*i.e.*, Fresh Ginger, *Sheng Jiang*), 2 slices

Method of preparation & administration: Cook the rice in water and make porridge as usual. Before the rice is completely cooked, add the powdered morning glory seeds and the ginger. Cook for a short time more. Each day, eat before noon on an empty stomach.

27
Diarrhea (*Xie Xie*)

Agastaches & Roasted Ginger Congee
(*Huo Xiang Wei Jiang Zhou*)

Functions: Relieves the exterior and courses wind, scatters cold and penetrates dampness

Indications: Cold damp or wind cold diarrhea

Ingredients: Herba Agastachis Seu Pogostemi (*Huo Xiang*), 6g, roasted Rhizoma Zingiberis (*Wei Jiang*), 6g, Radix Ledebouriellae

Sesloidis (*Fang Feng*), 3g, Fructus Cardamomi (*Bai Dou Kou Ren*), 3g, Semen Oryzae Sativae (*i.e.*, Polished Rice, *Jing Mi*), 100g

Method of preparation & administration: Decoct the first 4 ingredients in water, remove the dregs, and reserve the liquid. Then cook the rice in a suitable amount of water into porridge. When the porridge is almost cooked, add the medicinal liquid, mix thoroughly, and cook a few minutes more. Eat hot. Sweating after eating results in a cure.

Added Flavors Dry Ginger Congee
(*Jia Wei Gan Jiang Zhou*)

Functions: Warms the center and eliminates dampness

Indications: Cold damp diarrhea

Ingredients: Dry Rhizoma Zingiberis (*Gan Jiang*), 4.5g, Rhizoma Alpiniae Officinari (*Gao Liang Jiang*), 4.5g, Fructus Cardamomi (*Bai Dou Kou*), 3g, Semen Coicis Lachryma-jobi (*Yi Yi Ren*), 30g, Semen Oryzae Sativae (*i.e.*, Polished Rice, *Jing Mi*), 60g

Method of preparation & administration: Decoct the first 3 ingredients in water, remove the dregs, and reserve the liquid. Cook the rice and Coix into porridge using this liquid and eat 2 times per day.

Plantain & Dolichos Congee
(*Che Qian Bian Dou Zhou*)

Functions: Clears heat and eliminates dampness

Indications: Damp heat or summerheat diarrhea

Ingredients: Herba Plantaginis (*Che Qian Cao*), 15g, Herba Lophatheri Gracilis (*Dan Zhu Ye*), 9g, dry Folium Nelumbinis Nuciferae (*Gan He Ye*), 9g, Semen Dolichos Lablabis (*Bai Bian Dou*), 30g, Semen Coicis Lachryma-jobi (*Yi Mi Ren*), 30g, Semen Oryzae Sativae (*i.e.*, Polished Rice, *Jing Mi*), 60g

Method of preparation & administration: Decoct the first 3 ingredients, remove the dregs, and reserve the liquid. Make porridge out of the last 3 ingredients with a suitable amount of water. Just before the porridge is cooked, add the medicinal liquid and stir thoroughly, cooking the mixture a few minutes longer. Eat 2 times per day.

Powdered Kudzu Root Congee
(Ge Gen Fen Zhou)

Functions: Clears heat and eliminates vexation, engenders fluids and stops thirst, recedes rashes, and stops diarrhea, reduces blood pressure

Indications: Vexatious thirst due to febrile disease, macular rashes which do not recede, high blood pressure, diabetes mellitus in the elderly, chronic spleen vacuity diarrhea and dysentery, summertime thirst and desire for many cold drinks

Ingredients: Powdered Radix Puerariae Lobatae (*Ge Gen Fen*), 30g, Semen Oryzae Sativae (*i.e.*, Polished Rice, *Jing Mi*), 50g

Method of preparation & administration: First soak the rice in water overnight. Then cook the rice and kudzu root powder in 500ml of water and make into porridge. Eat warm at no fixed times.

Lotus Seed & Coix Congee
(Lian Yi Zhou)

Functions: Fortifies the spleen and dispels dampness

Indications: Spleen vacuity diarrhea, clear, watery stools, consumption and debility of fluids and humors, oral thirst, desire for drinks, etc.

Ingredients: Semen Nelumbinis Nuciferae (*Bai Lian Rou*), 30g, Semen Coicis Lachryma-jobi (*Yi Yi Ren*), 30g, Semen Oryzae Sativae (*i.e.*, Polished Rice, *Jing Mi*), 50g

Method of preparation & administration: Soak the lotus seeds and remove their skins. Then add the other 2 ingredients and cook into porridge. Divide into several portions and eat warm each time.

Jujube & Millet Congee
(Zao Su Zhou)

Functions: Boosts the spleen and stomach, stops diarrhea

Indications: Spleen and stomach vacuity heat resulting in diarrhea

Ingredients: Fructus Zizyphi Jujubae (*Da Zao*), 10 pieces, Semen Setariae Italicae (*i.e.*, Millet, *Su Zi*), 250g, Sclerotium Poriae Cocos (*Fu Ling*), 20g, Semen Oryzae Sativae (*i.e.*, Polished Rice, *Jing Mi*), 100g, White Sugar (*Bai Tang*), 30g

Method of preparation & administration: Make into porridge as usual. Add the sugar at the end and eat.

Cooked Rice Congee
(Jiao Mi Zhou)

Functions: Boosts the spleen and stomach, stops diarrhea

Indications: Spleen vacuity diarrhea, indigestion, watery diarrhea or pale, loose stools occurring too many times per day, no desire for food or drink

Ingredients: Polished Rice (*Bai Jing Mi*), 100g

Method of preparation & administration: First stir-fry the rice. Then add water and cook into porridge. It is ok to eat this as one pleases.

Chinese Yam & Egg Yolk Congee
(Shan Yao Ji Dan Zhou)

Functions: Fortifies the spleen and stomach and stops diarrhea

Indications: Diarrhea enduring many days, slippery intestines failing to secure

Ingredients: Radix Dioscoreae Oppositae (*Shan Yao*), 50g, Egg Yolk (*Ji Dan Huang*), 2 whole ones

Method of preparation & administration: First grind up the Chinese yam. Then add a suitable amount of water and bring to a boil 2-3 times. Add the egg yolks. Take 3 times per day on an empty stomach.

Litchi & Rice Congee
(Li Zhi Da Mi Zhou)

Functions: Fortifies the spleen and stops diarrhea

Indications: Chronic diarrhea or loose stools in the elderly

Ingredients: Dry Fructus Litchi Sinensis (*Gan Li Zhi*), 15 pieces, Radix Dioscoreae Oppositae (*Shan Yao*) and Semen Nelumbinis Nuciferae (*Lian Zi*), 15g each, Semen Oryzae Sativae (*i.e.*, Polished Rice, *Da Mi*), 50g

Method of preparation & administration: First decoct the first 3 ingredients. Remove the dregs and reserve the liquid. In this liquid, cook the rice into porridge and eat.

Lotus Seed & Rice Congee
(Lian Zi Jing Mi Zhou)

Functions: Fortifies the spleen and supplements vacuity

Indications: Spleen vacuity diarrhea, devitalized appetite for food and drink

Ingredients: Semen Nelumbinis Nuciferae (*Lian Zi*, without the center), 20g, Radix Dioscoreae Oppositae (*Shan Yao*), 25g, Endothelium Corneum Gigeriae Galli (*Ji Nei Jin*), 15g, Semen Oryzae Sativae (*i.e.*, Polished Rice, *Jing Mi*), 50g, White Sugar (*Bai Tang*), a suitable amount

Method of preparation & administration: Decoct the first 3 ingredients in water for 20 minutes. Then add the rice and make into porridge. After cooking, add the sugar and eat.

Pork Tripe & Rice Congee (*Zhu Du Da Mi Zhou*)

Functions: Supplements and boosts the spleen and stomach

Indications: Spleen/stomach vacuity diarrhea, polyuria

Ingredients: Pork Tripe (*Zhu Du*), 1 whole one, Radix Dioscoreae Oppositae (*Shan Yao*), 50g, Semen Oryzae Sativae (*i.e.*, Polished Rice, *Da Mi*), 50g, Salt (*Yan*) and Ginger (*Jiang*), each a suitable amount

Method of preparation & administration: Cut the pork tripe into pieces. Then add it and the Chinese yam to the rice and cook into porridge. Add some salt and ginger to taste.

Radish Seed & Hawthorne Berry Congee (*Lai Fu Shan Zha Zhou*)

Functions: Moves the food and disperses accumulation

Indications: Acute diarrhea due to overeating

Ingredients: Semen Raphani Sativi (*Lai Fu Zi*), 15g, Fructus Crataegi (*Shan Zha*), 20g, fresh Rhizoma Zingiberis (*i.e.*, Fresh Ginger, *Sheng Jiang*), 3 slices, Red Sugar (*i.e.*, Brown Sugar, *Hong Tang*), 15g, Semen Oryzae Sativae (*i.e.*, Polished Rice, *Da Mi*), 250g

Method of preparation & administration: First decoct the radish seeds, hawthorne berries, and ginger in a suitable amount of water for 40 minutes. Remove the dregs and reserve the liquid. Then cook the rice into porridge using this liquid. While still hot, add the brown sugar to flavor. Each day divide into 3 portions and eat. It is ok to do this 5 days in a row.

Aduki Bean & Chinese Yam Congee
(*Chi Xiao Dou Shan Yao Zhou*)

Functions: Supplements the spleen, clears heat, disinhibits dampness, stops diarrhea

Indications: Loss of spleen transportation with dampness smoldering and transforming into heat resulting in loose stools and short, scant urination, abdominal distention, heart vexation, oral thirst, etc.

Ingredients: Semen Phaseoli Calcarati (*i.e.*, Aduki Beans, *Chi Xiao Dou*), 50g, fresh Radix Dioscoreae Oppositae (*Xian Shan Yao*), 50g, White Sugar (*Bai Tang*), a suitable amount

Method of preparation & administration: First cook the aduki beans in water until half done. Then add the Chinese yam and cook till finished. Add sugar to taste and eat each morning.

Millet & Chinese Yam Congee
(*Su Mi Shan Yao Zhou*)

Functions: Fortifies the spleen and stomach, supplements the qi and blood

Indications: Spleen/stomach vacuity weakness resulting in diarrhea which may eventually lead to generalized qi and blood vacuity

Ingredients: Semen Setariae Italicae (*i.e.*, Millet, *Su Mi*), 50g, Radix Dioscoreae Oppositae (*Shan Yao*), 25g, Fructus Zizyphi Jujubae (*Da Zao*), 5 pieces

Method of preparation & administration: Make into porridge as usual and eat.

Chinese Yam & Jujube Congee
(*Shan Yao Da Zao Zhou*)

Functions: Supplements and boosts the spleen and stomach

Indications: Spleen vacuity, stomach weakness leading to chronic diarrhea, enduring diarrhea unable to be cured, occasionally occurs, occasionally stops, loose stools, lack of strength of the four limbs

Ingredients: Radix Dioscoreae Oppositae (*Shan Yao*), 30g, Fructus Zizyphi Jujubae (*Da Zao*), 10 pieces, Semen Coicis Lachryma-jobi (*Yi Mi*), 20g, Semen Oryzae Glutinosae (*i.e.*, Glutinous Rice, *Nuo Mi*), 30g, dry Rhizoma Zingiberis (*Gan Jiang*), 3 slices, Red Sugar (*i.e.*, Brown Sugar, *Hong Tang*), 15g

Method of preparation & administration: Make into porridge as usual. Each day divide into 3 portions and take. If one takes this continuously, they should heal in 1/2 month.

Chinese Yam, Lotus Seed & Euryales Congee
(*Shan Yao Lian Qian Zhou*)

Functions: Fortifies the spleen and eliminates dampness

Indications: Spleen qi vacuity and dampness diarrhea

Ingredients: Radix Dioscoreae Oppositae (*Shan Yao*), 15g, Semen Euryalis Ferocis (*Qian Shi*), 15g, Semen Nelumbinis Nuciferae (*Lian Zi*), 15g, Semen Dolichos Lablabis (*Bai Bian Dou*), 15g, Semen Coicis Lachryma-jobi (*Yi Yi Ren*), 15g, Fructus Zizyphi Jujubae (*Da Zao*), 10 pieces, Semen Oryzae Sativae (*i.e.*, Polished Rice, *Jing Mi*), 75g

Method of preparation & administration: Make into porridge as usual with all the above ingredients and eat 2 times per day.

Chinese Yam & Plantain Seed Congee
(*Shan Yao Che Qian Ze Zhou*)

Functions: Fortifies the spleen and secures the intestines, boosts the kidneys and disinhibits urination

Indications: Spleen/kidney vacuity leading to slippery, loose stools and inhibited urination

Ingredients: Fresh Radix Dioscoreae Oppositae (*Sheng Shan Yao*), 30g, Semen Plantaginis (*Che Qian Zi*), 12g

Method of preparation & administration: First grind the Chinese Yam into a fine powder and mix in cool water. Then add the plantain seeds wrapped in a bag and cook into porridge. Eat at no fixed times.

Alpinia Oxyphylla Congee
(*Yi Zhi Ren Zhou*)

Functions: Warms the center and stops diarrhea, supplements the kidneys and secures the essence

Indications: Spleen cold diarrhea, chilly pain within the abdomen, spermatorrhea, impotence, daybreak diarrhea, polyuria, urinary incontinence, nocturia

Ingredients: Semen Alpiniae Oxyphyllae (*Yi Zhi Ren*), 5g, Semen Oryzae Glutinosae (*i.e.*, Glutinous Rice, *Nuo Mi*), 50g, Salt (*Yan*), a small amount

Method of preparation & administration: Grind the Alpinia into fine powder. Then cook it, the rice, and water into porridge. Add salt to taste. Eat every day warm in the morning and evening.

Amomum Congee
(Sha Ren Zhou)

Functions: Transforms dampness and moves the qi, warms the spleen and stops diarrhea

Indications: Spleen/stomach vacuity cold abdominal pain, diarrhea, and dysentery, indigestion, epigastric and abdominal distention and fullness, devitalized appetite, restless fetus, nausea during pregnancy, qi counterflow (*i.e.*, hiccup) and vomiting

Ingredients: Powdered Fructus Amomi (*Sha Ren*) 5g, Semen Oryzae Sativae (*i.e.*, Polished Rice, *Da Mi*), 50g, Granulated Sugar (*Sha Tang*), a suitable amount

Method of preparation & administration: First cook the rice in 500ml of water into porridge. Then add the powdered Amomum and sugar and cook a short while longer. Eat warm in the morning and evening.

Added Flavors Cherokee Rose Hip Congee
(Jia Wei Jin Ying Zi Zhou)

Functions: Astringes the intestines and stops diarrhea

Indications: Enduring diarrhea due to kidney not securing and loss of astringency

Ingredients: Fructus Rosae Laevigatae (*Ji Ying Zi*), 12g, blast-fried Rhizoma Zingiberis (*Pao Jiang*), 6g, Semen Myristicae Fragrantis (*Rou Dou Kou*), 6g, Fructus Schizandrae Chinensis (*Wu Wei Zi*), 3g, Semen Nelumbinis Nuciferae (*Lian Zi*), 15g, Semen Euryalis Ferocis (*Qian Shi*), 15g, Radix Dioscoreae Oppositae (*Shan Yao*), 15g, Semen Oryzae Sativae (*i.e.*, Polished Rice, *Jing Mi*), 50g

Method of preparation & administration: Decoct the first 4 ingredients, remove the dregs, and reserve the liquid. Then make porridge with the last 4 ingredients and a suitable amount of water. Just before the porridge is done, add the reserved medicinal liquid and mix thoroughly, cooking a few minutes more. Eat 2 times per day.

Blast-fried Ginger Congee
(Pao Jiang Zhou)

Functions: Warms the center and stops diarrhea

Indications: Invasion of cold and dampness resulting in diarrhea, clear, watery stools, abdominal distention and fullness, lack of strength of the four limbs

Ingredients: Blast-fried Rhizoma Zingiberis (*Pao Jiang*), 6g, Rhizoma Atractylodis Macrocephalae (*Bai Zhu*), 15g, Fructus Zanthoxyli Bungeani (*i.e.*, Sichuan Pepper, *Hua Jiao*), a small amount, Semen Oryzae Glutinosae (*i.e.*, Glutinous Rice, *Nuo Mi*), 30g

Method of preparation & administration: Decoct the first 3 ingredients first for 20 minutes. Then add the rice and cook into porridge. Each day divide into 3 portions and eat. Take continuosly for 1-2 weeks.

Added Flavors Aconite Congee
(Jia Wei Fu Zi Zhou)

Functions: Supplements spleen/kidney yang

Indications: Enduring diarrhea due to spleen/kidney yang vacuity

Ingredients: Radix Praeparatus Aconiti Carmichaeli (*Zhi Fu Zi*), 6g, blast-fried Rhizoma Zingiberis (*Pao Jiang*), 6g, Semen Myristicae Fragrantis (*Rou Dou Kou*), 6g, Fructus Psoraleae Corylifoliae (*Bu Gu Zhi*), 6g, Sclerotium Poriae Cocos (*Fu Ling*), 15g, Semen Oryzae Sativae (*i.e.*, Polished Rice, *Jing Mi*), 100g, Red Sugar (*i.e.*, Brown Sugar, *Hong Tang*), a suitable amount

Method of preparation & administration: Decoct the first 5 ingredients, remove the dregs, and reserve the liquid. Add the rice and more water to this liquid and cook into porridge. When the porridge is cooked, add the brown sugar and eat 2 times per day.

Fresh Bamboo Shoot Congee
(Xian Zhu Sun Zhou)

Functions: Cools the blood and stops diarrhea

Indications: Enduring diarrhea, enduring dysentery, anal prolapse

Ingredients: Fresh Bamboo Shoot (*Xian Zhu Sun*), 1 whole piece, Semen Oryzae Sativae (*i.e.*, Polished Rice, *Da Mi*), 100g

Method of preparation & administration: Remove the skin from the bamboo shoot and cut into pieces. Add to the rice and cook into porridge. Take 1 time each morning and evening.

28
Dysentery (Li Ji)

Purslane Congee
(Ma Chi Xian Zhou)

Functions: Clears heat and disinhibits dampness

Indications: Red and white dysentery, tenesmus, epigastric and abdominal distention and fullness

Ingredients: Herba Portulacae Oleraceae (*Ma Chi Xian*), 500g, Semen Oryzae Sativae (*i.e.*, Polished Rice, *Jing Mi*), 100g

Method of preparation & administration: First wash the purslane. Then mash and press out the juice. Add this to the rice and cook into porridge. Take on an empty stomach.

Sophora Flower Congee
(Huai Hua Zhou)

Functions: Clears heat and resolves toxins, eliminates dampness, stops bleeding

Indications: Lower burner bleeding including hemafecia and hematuria, bloody dysentery, bleeding hemorrhoids

Ingredients: Dry Flos Immaturus Sophorae Japonicae (*Gan Huai Hua*), 30g, Semen Oryzae Sativae (*i.e.*, Polished Rice, *Da Mi*), 50g

Method of preparation & administration: Make the rice into porridge as usual. Then add the Sophora flowers and continue cooking for some time. Afterwards eat.

White Wood Ear Congee
(Bai Mu Er Zhou)

Functions: Enriches yin and moistens dryness

Indications: Enduring dysentery damaging yin, dry mouth and throat

Ingredients: White Fructificatio Tremellae (*Bai Mu Er*, a.k.a. *Yin Er*) 50g, Semen Oryzae Sativae (*i.e.*, Polished Rice, *Jing Mi*), 50g, Succus Semenis Praeparati Sojae, (*i.e.*, Fermented Soybean Juice, *Chi Zhi*), Bulbus Alli Fistulosi (*i.e.*, Scallion, *Cong*), Pepper (*Jiao*), Salt (*Yan*), each a suitable amount

Method of preparation & administration: Soak the tree ears and cut into pieces. Boil the first 3 ingredients into porridge. Afterwards, add the scallion, pepper, salt, etc. to taste. Take on an empty stomach.

Turtle Egg Congee
(Gui Dan Zhou)

Functions: Stops bleeding and diarrhea

Indications: Red and white dysentery

Ingredients: Turtle Egg (*Gui Dan*), 1 whole one, Semen Oryzae Sativae (*i.e.*, Polished Rice, *Jing Mi*), 50g

Method of preparation & administration: First make porridge as usual out of the rice. Then crack the egg and stir the contents into the porridge. Continue cooking briefly and eat.

Quail & Aduki Bean Congee (*An Chun Chi Dou Zhou*)

Functions: Supplements the five viscera, stops downward dysentery

Indications: Red and white dysentery. This is also a very enriching and nourishing food.

Ingredients: Quail (*An Chun*), 1 piece, Semen Phaseoli Calcarati (*i.e.*, Aduki Beans, *Chi Xiao Dou*), 30g, fresh Rhizoma Zingiberis (*i.e.*, fresh Ginger, *Xian Jiang*), 5 slices

Method of preparation & administration: Remove the skin and guts from the quail and cut into chunks. then cook together with the aduki beans and ginger into porridge. Eat 2 times per day.

Three Treasures Congee (*San Bao Zhou*)

Functions: Fortifies the spleen and secures the intestines, resolves toxins and stops dysentery

Indications: Stagnant heat smoldering internally leading to downward dysentery which does not stop, pus and blood in the stools, abdominal pain and distention, tenesmus, and simultaneous signs and symptoms of spleen qi vacuity weakness such as lack of strength, emaciation, poor appetite, etc.

Ingredients: Fresh Radix Dioscoreae Oppositae (*Sheng Shan Yao*), 30g, powdered Radix Pseudoginseng (*San Qi*), 6g, Duck Eggs (*Ya Dan Zi*), 2 whole ones without the shell

Method of preparation & administration: First grind the Chinese yam into a fine powder and cook in water into porridge. Bring to a boil 3 times and then add the Pseudoginseng and duck eggs. Eat each morning.

Tea Leaf Congee
(*Cha Ye Zhou*)

Functions: Strengthens the heart, disinhibits water, attacks germs, resolves toxins, transforms phlegm, and disperses food

Indications: Acute and chronic dysentery, colitis, acute and chronic gastritis, amebic dysentery, water swelling due to heart disease, pulmonary heart disease, water swelling due to nephritis, urinary tract infection, stomach and duodenal ulcers, high blood pressure, cholecystitis

Ingredients: Folium Camelliae Theae (*i.e.*, Tea Leaves, *Cha Ye*), 10g, Semen Oryzae Sativae (*i.e.*, Polished Rice, *Jing Mi*), 50g, White Sugar (*Bai Tang*), a suitable amount

Method of preparation & administration: First steep the tea leaves in 100ml of boiling water. Remove the leaves and add to the rice along with 400ml more water. Cook into porridge as usual. Add sugar to taste and eat warm 2 times per day.

Contraindications: Insomnia, habitual constipation. Breast-feeding women should not use this congee. This congee should also not be used at the same time as taking Ginseng or blood-supplementing medicinals.

29
Constipation (*Bian Bi*)

Prune Seed Congee
(*Yu Li Ren Zhou*)

Functions: Moistens the intestines and frees the stools, disinhibits water and disperses swelling

Indications: Large intestine qi stagnation, intestinal dryness constipation, possible foot qi and superficial edema, inhibited urination

Ingredients: Semen Pruni (*Yu Li Ren*), 10g, Semen Oryzae Sativae (*i.e.*, Polished Rice, *Jing Mi*), 100g, Honey (*Mi Tang*) and fresh Ginger Juice (*Sheng Jiang Zhi*), each a suitable amount

Method of preparation & administration: Soak the prune seeds and remove the skin. Mash into a paste. Cook the rice into porridge and then add the prune seed mash, ginger juice, and honey. Eat on an empty stomach.

Perilla Seed Congee
(*Su Zi Zhou*)

Functions: Clears the lungs, moistens the intestines, engenders fluids

Indications: Dry constipation in the elderly, qi vacuity coughing and panting

Ingredients: Purple Fructus Perillae Frutescentis (*Zi Su Zi*), 15g, White Fructus Perillae Frutescentis (*Bai Su Zi*), 15g, Semen Oryzae Sativae (*i.e.*, Polished Rice, *Jing Mi*), 30g. (Li Shi-zhen distinguished between a purple and a white Perilla. In this case, 15g of each variety is used.)

Method of preparation & administration: Stir-fry the white Perilla seeds. Then grind both Perilla seeds into a pulpy mash and boil this in water. Press out the juice and use this to cook the rice into porridge. One may also add ginger juice or a little honey to taste.

Pine Nut Congee
(Song Ren Zhou)

Functions: Enriches yin and moistens the lungs, moistens the intestines and frees the stool

Indications: Fluid dryness constipation in the weak, elderly, or postpartum, dry cough with phlegm, dry throat, dry skin, etc.

Ingredients: Semen Pini (*i.e.*, Pine Nuts, *Song Zi Ren*), 30g, Semen Oryzae Glutinosae (*i.e.*, Glutinous Rice, *Nuo Mi*), 50g, Honey (*Mi Tang*), a suitable amount

Method of preparation & administration: Add 400ml of water and cook into porridge adding the honey at the end. Take warm on an empty stomach, 2 times per day, morning and evening.

Contraindications: Do not use in case of spleen/stomach vacuity weakness loose stools or diarrhea, excessive phlegm, stomach and epigastric distention and fullness, vomiting, devitalized appetite, etc.

Cistanches Congee
(Rou Cong Rong Zhou)

Functions: Supplements the kidneys and strengthens yang, moistens the intestines and frees the stools

Indications: Yang vacuity constipation, kidney life gate fire debility, lack of warmth in the four limbs, low back and knee chilly pain, etc.

Ingredients: Herba Cistanchis (*Rou Cong Rong*), 15g, Lamb (*Yang Rou*), 50g, Semen Oryzae Sativae (*i.e.*, Polished Rice, *Jing Mi*), 100g

Method of preparation & administration: First decoct the Cistanches and cut up the lamb meat. Remove the dregs from the Cistanches decoction and reserve the liquid. Add this liquid and the lamb to the rice and cook into porridge. Eat on an empty stomach.

Three Seed Congee
(San Ren Zhou)

Functions: Moistens the intestines, dispels wind, stops pain

Indications: Wind constipation. This condition typically occurs in the elderly and is accompanied by headache and abdominal pain, no desire for food or drink, chest and abdominal distention and fullness, dry, knotted stools

Ingredients: Semen Pini Koraiensis (*Hai Song Zi*), 30g, Semen Pruni Persicae (*Tao Ren*), 30g, Semen Pruni (*Yu Li Ren*), 10g, Semen Oryzae Sativae (*i.e.*, Polished Rice, *Jing Mi*), 30g

Method of preparation & administration: Remove the skin from these 3 seeds and the tip from the peach seeds. Grind them into a mash and boil in water. Then add to the rice and cook into porridge. Eat on an empty stomach.

Note: One may substitute Pine Nuts for the Semen Pini Koraiensis.

Cow's Milk Congee
(Niu Ru Zhou)

Functions: Supplements vacuity detriment, boosts the lungs and stomach, engenders fluids and humors, moistens intestinal dryness

Indications: Vacuity, weakness, taxation, and detriment, poor nutrition, anemia, bodily vacuity weakness after disease or postpartum, vacuity constipation in the elderly

Ingredients: Cow's Milk (*Niu Ru*), 200ml, either Semen Oryzae Sativae (*i.e.*, Polished Rice, *Jing Mi*) or Semen Oryzae Glutinosae (*i.e.*, Glutinous Rice, *Nuo Mi*), 100g

Method of preparation & administration: Add these two ingredients to 500ml of water and cook into porridge. One may add a small amount of White Sugar (*Bai Tang*) to taste. Eat daily on an empty stomach.

30
Kidney Vacuity Urinary Incontinence
(*Shen Xu Yi Niao*)

Allium Seed Congee
(*Jiu Cai Zi Zhou*)

Functions: Supplements the kidneys and strengthens yang, secures the essence and stops loss

Indications: Kidney vacuity urinary incontinence, spermatorrhea

Ingredients: Semen Allii Tuberosi (*i.e.*, Chinese Chive Seeds, *Jiu Cai Zi*), 25g, Polished Rice (*Da Mi*), 100g

Method of preparation & administration: Cook into porridge as usual and eat 1 time per day.

31
Acute & Chronic Nephritis,
Renal Tuberculosis
(*Ji Man Xing Shen Yan, Shen Jie He*)

Carp & Juncus Congee
(*Ji Yu Deng Xin Zhou*)

Functions: Regulates the stomach, fills the intestines, descends the qi

Indications: Chronic nephritis, intestinal wind with hemafecia

Ingredients: Crucian Carp (*Ji Yu*), 1-2 pieces, Medulla Junci Effusi (*Deng Xin Cao*), 7-8 roots, Semen Oryzae Sativae (*i.e.*, Polished Rice, *Da Mi*), 50g

Method of preparation & administration: First remove the scales and the guts. Then cook the carp and the Juncus together in water. Later, remove the dregs and add to the rice. Cook into porridge and eat.

Shepherd's Purse Congee
(*Ji Cai Zhou*)

Functions: Boosts the qi, fortifies the spleen, brightens the eyes, and stops bleeding

Indications: Chronic nephritis, vacuity weakness in the elderly, water swelling, chyluria, hemoptysis, hematemesis, hemafecia, hematuria, etc.

Ingredients: Fresh Herba Capsellae Bursa-pastoris (*i.e.*, Shepherd's Purse, *Xian Ji Cai*), 250g, Semen Oryzae Sativae (*i.e.*, Polished Rice, *Jing Mi*), 100g

Method of preparation & administration: Cook into porridge in water as usual. Eat warm 2 times per day.

Astragalus Congee with Added Flavors
(*Huang Qi Zhou Jia Wei*)

Functions: Supplements the qi, disinhibits water, rectifies the qi

Indications: Water swelling due to chronic nephritis and pyelonephritis, chyluria associated with chronic nephritis

Ingredients: Fresh Radix Astragali Membranacei (*Sheng Huang Qi*), Semen Coicis Lachryma-jobi (*Yi Yi Ren*), Semen Oryzae Glutinosae (*i.e.*, Glutinous Rice, *Nuo Mi*), 30g each, Semen Phaseoli Calcarati (*i.e.*, Aduki Beans, *Chi Xiao Dou*), 15g, Endothelium Corneum Gigeriae Galli (*Ji Nei Jin*), 9g, Pericarpium Citri Reticulatae (*Chen Pi*), 3g

Method of preparation & administration: First decoct the Astragalus and orange peel in 600ml of water for 20 minutes. Remove the dregs and reserve the liquid. Add the Coix and aduki beans and cook for 30 minutes. Powder the chicken gizzard membrane and add it and the glutinous rice and cook into porridge. Eat daily in 2 divided doses.

32
Strangury Diseases (*Lin Bing*)

Millet Congee
(*Xiao Mi Zhou*)

Functions: Clears evil heat, disinhibits urination

Indications: Damp heat of the spleen, stomach, and kidneys leading to urinary dribbling and dripping

Ingredients: Semen Setariae Italicae (*i.e.*, Millet, *Xiao Mi*), 100g

Method of preparation & administration: Cook into porridge as usual and eat.

Small Green Bean Congee
(*Qing Xiao Dou Zhou*)

Functions: Clears heat and disinhibits dampness

Indications: Acute cystitis

Ingredients: Semen Phaseoli Mungonis (*i.e.*, Mung Beans, *Lu Dou*), 50g, Medulla Tetrapanacis Papyriferi (*Tong Cao*), 10g, Fructus Tritici (*i.e.*, Wheat, *Xiao Mai*), 50g

Method of preparation & administration: First decoct the Tetrapanax in 2,000ml of water and reduce to 1,000ml. Remove the dregs and reserve the liquid. Then cook the mung beans and wheat in this liquid into porridge and eat.

Aduki Bean & Chicken Gizzard Membrane Congee (*Chi Xiao Dou Nei Jin Zhou*)

Functions: Clears heat and disinhibits dampness, transforms stones

Indications: Acute cystitis, kidney and bladder stones

Ingredients: Semen Phaseoli Calcarati (*i.e.*, Aduki Beans, *Chi Xiao Dou*), a suitable amount, powdered Endothelium Corneum Gigeriae Galli (*Ji Nei Jin Fen*), a suitable amount

Method of preparation & administration: Cook the aduki beans into porridge and add the chicken gizzard membrane powder just before done. Cook for a few minutes more and eat.

Malva Verticillata Congee (*Kui Cai Zhou*)

Functions: Clears heat and disinhibits dampness

Indications: Acute cystitis

Ingredients: Herba Malvae Verticillatae (*Kui Cai*), 200g, Bulbus Allii Fistulosi (*i.e.*, Scallion, *Cong Bai*), 3 stalks, Semen Oryzae Sativae (*i.e.*, Polished Rice, *Jing Mi*), Fermented Soybean Juice (*Nong Chi Ye*), a small amount

Method of preparation & administration: First decoct the Malva, remove the dregs, and reserve the liquid. Use this liquid to cook the rice and scallion into a porridge. When the porridge is done, add some fermented soybean juice and mix thoroughly. Eat on an empty stomach.

Talcum Congee
(Hua Shi Zhou)

Functions: Clears heat and percolates dampness

Indications: All types of acute urinary tract infections due to damp heat.

Ingredients: Talcum (*Hua Shi*, wrapped in a cloth bag), 30g, Herba Dianthi (*Qu Mai*), 10g, Semen Oryzae Sativae (*i.e.*, Polished Rice, *Jing Mi*), 50g

Method of preparation & administration: Decoct the first 2 ingredients, remove the dregs, and reserve the liquid. Then cook the rice in this liquid into porridge and eat.

Contraindications: Pregnant women should not use this congee.

Bamboo Leaf Congee
(Zhu Ye Zhou)

Functions: Clears heat and percolates dampness

Indications: Urinary problems due to damp heat in the lower burner

Ingredients: Fresh Folium Bambusae (*Xian Zhu Ye*), 30g, Gypsum Fibrosum (*Shi Gao*), 60g, Semen Oryzae Sativae (*i.e.*, Polished Rice, *Jing Mi*), 100g

Method of preparation & administration: First decoct the bamboo leaves and Gypsum, remove the dregs, and reserve the liquid. Cook the rice in this liquid into porridge and eat.

Coix & Prune Seed Congee
(Yi Mi Yu Li Zhou)

Functions: Clears heat, eliminates dampness, quickens the blood and dispels stasis

Indications: Prostatic hypertrophy and urinary strangury due to damp heat and qi and blood stagnation and stasis in the lower burner

Ingredients: Semen Coicis Lachryma-jobi (Yi Mi), a suitable amount, Semen Pruni (Yu Li), a suitable amount

Method of preparation & administration: Make into porridge as usual and eat.

Cinnamon Congee
(Gui Xin Zhou)

Functions: Warms yang and returns it to its lower origin

Indications: Urinary strangury and prostatic hypertrophy due to decline of life gate fire, impotence

Ingredients: Powdered Cortex Cinnamomi (Gui Xin Fen), a suitable amount, Semen Oryzae Sativae (i.e., Polished Rice, Jing Mi), 60g

Method of preparation & administration: Cook the rice into porridge and sprinkle on a suitable amount of powdered cinnamon. Mix thoroughly and eat 2 times per day.

Chinese Chive Congee
(Jiu Cai Zhou)

Functions: Supplements the spleen and kidneys and warms yang

Indications: Qi and yang vacuity urinary strangury and prostatic hypertrophy

Ingredients: Herba Allii Tuberosi (i.e., Chinese Chive, Jiu Cai), a suitable amount, Polished Rice (Jing Mi), a suitable amount

Method of preparation & administration: Make these into porridge as usual and eat.

33
Impotence (*Yang Wei*)

Deer Kidney Congee
(*Lu Shen Zhou*)

Functions: Boosts the kidneys and strengthens yang

Indications: Kidney vacuity deafness and tinnitus, low back soreness, weak lower legs, lack of strength

Ingredients: Deer Kidney (*Lu Shen*), 1 pair, Semen Oryzae Sativae (*i.e.*, Polished Rice, *Jing Mi*), 100g, fresh Rhizoma Zingiberis (*i.e.*, Ginger, *Jiang*), Herba Alli Fistulosi (*i.e.*, Scallion, *Cong*), Salt (*Yan*), a small amount

Method of preparation & administration: Cut open the deer kidneys and remove the membranes. Then cut into pieces and cook with the rice into porridge. Add ginger, scallions, and salt to taste. Eat on an empty stomach.

Note: If 30g of Herba Cistanchis (*Rou Cong Rong*) are added, this congee then treats impotence and inability to achieve an erection.

Five Flavors Congee
(*Wu Wei Zhou*)

Functions: Supplements the kidneys and boosts the essence, assists yang affairs

Indications: Treats impotence, lack of strength in the low back and lower legs, the five consumptions and seven damages in males, and kidney vacuity conditions

Ingredients: Lamb Kidneys (*Yang Yao Zi*), 3 pair, Lamb (*Yang Rou*), 250g, Bulbus Allii Fistulosi (*i.e.*, Scallion, *Cong Bai*), 1 root, Folium Lycii Chinensis (*Gou Qi Ye*), 500g, Semen Oryzae Sativae (*i.e.*, Polished Rice, *Da Mi*), 100g

Method of preparation & administration: First remove all the sinews and membranes from the lamb kidneys and cut into pieces. Wash the lamb meat and also cut into pieces. Likewise, cut up the scallion bulb. Wash both the Lycium leaves and the rice. Then cook all of these together into porridge and eat 1 time per day.

Cuscuta Congee
(*Tu Si Zi Zhou*)

Functions: Enriches and supplements the liver and kidneys

Indications: Liver/kidney insufficiency, impotence, spermatorrhea, premature ejaculation, low back and knee sinew and bone pain, foot and lower leg weakness and lack of strength, polyuria, dizziness, blurred vision, diminished visual acuity, deafness, tinnitus, abnormal vaginal discharge in women, habitual miscarriage

Ingredients: Ground Semen Cuscutae (*Tu Si Zi*), 60g, Semen Oryzae Sativae (*i.e.*, Polished Rice, *Jing Mi*), 100g, White Sugar (*Bai Tang*), a suitable amount

Method of preparation & administration: First decoct the Cuscuta in 300ml of water down to 200ml, remove the dregs, and reserve the liquid. Add this and 800ml more water to the rice and cook into porridge as usual. Eat warm each morning and evening. Ten days equal 1 course of treatment.

Cynomorium Congee
(Suo Yang Zhou)

Functions: Supplements and boosts the liver and kidneys, moistens the intestines and frees the stool

Indications: Kidney vacuity impotence, spermatorrhea, sinew and bone atony and weakness, difficulty moving about, blood vacuity, fluid damage, and yin damage of the liver and kidneys, intestinal dryness constipation

Ingredients: Herba Cynomorii Songarici (*Suo Yang*), 30g, Semen Oryzae Sativae (*i.e.*, Polished Rice, *Da Mi*), 50g

Method of preparation & administration: Add water and cook into porridge as usual. Strain out the cynomorium. It is ok not to eat.

34
Spermatorrhea (Yi Jing)

Euryales Congee
(Qian Shi Zhou)

Functions: Secures the essence

Indications: Kidney qi not securing spermatorrhea

Ingredients: Semen Euryalis Ferocis (*Qian Shi*), a suitable amount, Exocarpium Fructi Tritici (*i.e.*, Wheat Bran, *Mai Fu*), a suitable amount, Semen Oryzae Sativae (*i.e.*, Polished Rice, *Jing Mi*), a suitable amount

Method of preparation & administration: Stir-fry the first 2 ingredients till yellow colored. Then take 15-20g of this mixture and boil with 30g of rice in 500ml of water over a slow fire until this thickens. Take warm, before meals, 2 times per day in the morning and evening.

Lotus Seed Congee
(*Lian Rou Zhou*)

Functions: Secures the essence

Indications: Kidney qi not securing spermatorrhea

Ingredients: Powdered Semen Nelumbinis Nuciferae (*Lian Zi Fen*), 15g, Semen Oryzae Glutinosae (*i.e.,* Glutinous Rice, *Nuo Mi*), 30g, Red Sugar (*i.e.*, Brown Sugar, *Hong Tang*), a suitable amount

Method of preparation & administration: Make into porridge as usual and eat 2 times per day in the morning and evening.

Cornus Congee
(*Shan Yu Rou Zhou*)

Functions: Supplements the kidneys and secures the essence, stops sweating

Indications: Spermatorrhea, spontaneous sweating, polyuria, low back and knee soreness and weakness, dizziness, deafness, tinnitus

Ingredients: Fructus Corni Officinalis (*Shan Zhu Yu*), 20g, Semen Oryzae Sativae (*i.e.*, Polished Rice, *Jing Mi*), 60g, White Sugar (*Bai Tang*), a suitable amount

Method of preparation & administration: Wash the Cornus and remove the pits. Add to the rice and cook into porridge as usual. Add sugar to taste and continue cooking for a few minutes more. Eat 2 times per day in the morning and evening.

35
Low Back & Knee Aching & Pain
(*Yao Xi Teng Tong*)

Lamb Bone & Millet Congee
(*Yang Gu Su Mi Zhou*)

Functions: Supplements the kidneys, strengthens and fortifies the sinews and bones, moistens dryness and dispels cold

Indications: Kidney vacuity low back pain, deafness, vacuity taxation and lack of strength conditions

Ingredients: Lamb Bone (*Yang Gu*), a suitable amount, Semen Setariae Italicae (*i.e.*, Millet, *Su Mi*), 100g, Pericarpium Citri Reticulatae (*Chen Pi*), 5g, fresh Rhizoma Zingiberis, (*i.e.*, Ginger, *Jiang*), 20g, Fructus Amomi Tsao-ko (*Cao Guo*), 2 whole ones, Salt (*Yan*), a small amount

Method of preparation & administration: Break open the lamb bone to expose the marrow. Remove the white from the orange peel. Decoct the ginger and Amomum Tsao-ko in water and remove the dregs. Then use this liquid to make a porridge with the rice and preceding ingredients. Add a little salt to taste and eat.

Chestnut & Rice Congee
(*Li Zi Da Mi Zhou*)

Functions: Supplements the kidneys and strengthens the sinews

Indications: Kidney vacuity leading to low back soreness and pain of the lower legs

Ingredients: Chestnuts (*Li Zi*), 100g, Semen Oryzae Sativae (*i.e.*, Polished Rice, *Da Mi*), 50g, White Sugar (*Bai Tang*), a suitable amount

Method of preparation & administration: Cook into porridge as usual. After cooking, mix in some sugar and take.

36
Kidney Egg Pain
(*i.e.., Testicular Pain & Swelling*)
(*Shen Zi Tong*)

Orange Seed Congee
(*Ju He Zhou*)

Functions: Moves the qi, scatters nodulation, stops pain

Indications: Testicular swelling, distention, and pain, *shan* qi swelling and pain, breast abscess

Ingredients: Semen Citri (*Ju He*), 10g, Semen Oryzae Sativae (*i.e.*, Polished Rice, *Jing Mi*), 50g

Method of preparation & administration: First decoct the orange seeds in water, then add the rice and more water and cook into porridge. Strain out the orange seeds and eat warm 2 times per day

37
Spontaneous Sweating, Night Sweats
(*Zi Han, Dao Han*)

Floating (*i.e.*, Blighted) Wheat Congee
(*Fu Xiao Mai Zhou*)

Functions: Boosts the qi, eliminates heat, and stops sweating

Indications: Spontaneous sweating, night sweats, women's taxation heat, steaming bone and vacuity heat

Ingredients: Powdered Semen Levis Tritici (*Fu Xiao Mai Fen*), 20g, Semen Oryzae Glutinosae (*i.e.*, Glutinous Rice, *Nuo Mi*), 50g

Method of preparation & administration: First cook the rice in water into porridge. Then add the powdered blighted wheat and continue cooking a few minutes more. Eat warm each morning and evening.

CHAPTER 2

GYNECOLOGY
(FU KE)

1
Menstrual Irregularity
(Yue Jing Shi Tiao)

Dang Gui Congee
(Dang Gui Zhou)

Functions: Supplements the blood and regulates the menses, quickens the blood and stops pain, moistens the intestines and frees the stool

Indications: Qi and blood insufficiency, menstrual irregularity, amenorrhea, dysmenorrhea, blood vacuity headache, dizziness and vertigo, blood vacuity constipation

Ingredients: Radix Angelicae Sinensis (*Dang Gui*), 15g, Fructus Ziziphi Jujubae (*Da Zao*), 5 pieces, Semen Oryzae Sativae (*i.e.*, Polished Rice, *Jing Mi*), 50g, Granulated Sugar (*Sha Tang*), a suitable amount

Method of preparation & administration: First decoct the Dang Gui in water, remove the dregs, and reserve 100ml of liquid. Add this to the rice, jujubes, and sugar plus 300ml more water and cook into porridge. Eat warm each morning and evening on an empty stomach. Ten days equal 1 course of treatment.

Motherwort Juice Congee
(Yi Mu Cao Zhi Zhou)

Functions: Nourishes and quickens the blood, stops bleeding

Indications: Irregular menstruation and excessive menstrual bleeding

Ingredients: Succus Herbae Leonuri Heterophylli (*i.e.*, Motherwort Juice, *Yi Mu Cao Zhi*), 10ml, Succus Radicis Rehmanniae (*i.e.*, Rehmannia Juice, *Sheng Di Huang Zhi*), 40ml, Succus Rhizomatis Nelumbinis Nuciferae (*i.e.*, Lotus Root Juice, *Ou Zhi*), Succus Rhizomatis Zingiberis (*i.e.*, Ginger Juice, *Sheng Jiang Zhi*), 2ml, Honey (*Mi Tang*), 10ml, Semen Oryzae Sativae (*i.e.*, Polished Rice, *Jing Mi*), 100g

Method of preparation & administration: First make a porridge out of the rice. Then add all the above juices and honey. Mix thoroughly and cook for a few minutes more.

2
Dysmenorrhea, Delayed Periods
(Tong Jing, Yue Jing Hou Qi)

Hawthorne Berry Congee
(Shan Zha Zhou)

Functions: Quickens the blood and transforms stasis

Indications: Dysmenorrhea and delayed periods due to stagnation and stasis

Ingredients: Fructus Crataegi (*Shan Zha*), 40g, Semen Oryzae Sativae (*i.e.*, Polished Rice, *Jing Mi*), 100g, Granulated Sugar (*Bing Tang*), 10g

Method of preparation & administration: Boil the hawthorne berries first into a thick decoction. Add this to the rice and sugar and make into porridge, adding as much water as necessary.

Allium Congee
(Xie Bai Zhou)

Functions: Moves the qi and quickens the blood

Indications: Dysmenorrhea due to qi stagnation, blood stasis

Ingredients: Bulbus Allii Macrostemi (*Xie Bai*), 10g, Semen Oryzae Sativae (*i.e.*, Polished Rice, *Jing Mi*), 50g

Method of preparation & administration: Make into porridge as usual and eat.

Mugwort Congee
(Ai Ye Zhou)

Functions: Warms the channels (menses) and stops bleeding, scatters cold and stops pain

Indications: Vacuity cold dysmenorrhea, menstrual irregularity, lower abdominal chilly pain, profuse uterine bleeding, restless fetus, cold uterus infertility

Ingredients: Dry Folium Artemisiae Argyii (*Gan Ai Ye*), 15g, Semen Oryzae Sativae (*i.e.*, Polished Rice, *Jing Mi*), 50g, Red Sugar (*i.e.*, Brown Sugar, *Hong Tang*), a suitable amount

Method of preparation & administration: First decoct the mugwort, remove the dregs, and reserve the liquid. Then cook the rice into porridge and add the medicinal liquid and sugar. Take beginning 3 days after the period ends and stop taking 3 days before it begins again. Each day eat 2 times, morning and evening, warm.

Salvia Congee
(Dan Shen Zhou)

Functions: Quickens the blood and transforms stasis, clears heat and soothes vexation, nourishes the heart and quiets the spirit

Indications: Stasis and stagnation abdominal pain, menstrual irregularity, blood stasis amenorrhea, postpartum lochia will not stop, infertility, chest and lateral costal aching and pain

Ingredients: Radix Salviae Miltiorrhizae (*Dan Shen*), 30g, Semen Oryzae Glutinosae (*i.e.*, Glutinous Rice, *Nuo Mi*), 50g, Fructus Zizyphi Jujubae (*Hong Zao*), 3 pieces, Red Sugar (*i.e.*, Brown Sugar, *Hong Tang*), a suitable amount

Method of preparation & administration: First decoct the Salvia in water, remove the dregs, and reserve the liquid. Add the rice, jujubes, and sugar and cook into porridge as usual. Eat warm 2 times per day. Ten days equals 1 course of treatment. Rest 3 days before beginning again.

Motherwort Congee
(Yi Mu Cao Zhou)

Functions: Moves and nourishes the blood, moves the blood without injuring fresh or new blood

Indications: Dysmenorrhea, menstrual irregularity, leaking fetus, difficult delivery, profuse uterine bleeding, postpartum blood dizziness, static blood abdominal pain, etc.

Ingredients: Dry Herba Leonuri Heterophyllae (*Gan Yi Mu Cao*), 60g, Semen Oryzae Sativae (*i.e.*, Polished Rice, *Jing Mi*), 50g, Red Sugar (*i.e.*, Brown Sugar, *Hong Tang*), a suitable amount

Method of preparation & administration: First decoct the motherwort, remove the dregs, and reserve the liquid. This should amount to approximately 200ml. Add this to the rice, sugar, and another 300ml of water and cook into porridge. Take 2 times per day warm.

Chicken Broth Congee
(Ji Zhi Zhou)

Functions: Nourishes the five viscera and supplements the qi and blood

Indications: Dysmenorrhea due to qi and blood vacuity, postpartum vacuity weakness

Ingredients: Female Chicken (*Mu Ji*), 1, Semen Oryzae Sativae (*i.e.*, Polished Rice, *Jing Mi*), 100g

Method of preparation & administration: Boil a chicken in water until it falls apart. Strain out this soupy extract, skim off the fat, and reserve. Then make porridge from the rice and water. When the porridge is almost done, add this soupy extract and continue cooking for a few minutes more. Then eat.

Lamb Congee
(Yang Rou Zhou)

Functions: Supplements the qi and blood

Indications: Dysmenorrhea due to qi and blood vacuity

Ingredients: Lamb (*Yang Rou*), 100g, Semen Sorghi Vulgaris (*i.e.*, Husked Sorghum, *Gao Liang*), 100g

Method of preparation & administration: Make a porridge with the lamb and rice as usual. Season with scallion and salt to taste.

3
Amenorrhea (*Jing Bi*)

Peach Seed Congee
(*Tao Ren Zhou*)

Functions: Quickens the blood and dispels stasis

Indications: Amenorrhea and dysmenorrhea due to blood stasis

Ingredients: Semen Pruni Persicae (*Tao Ren*), 15g, Semen Oryzae Sativae (*i.e.*, Polished Rice, *Jing Mi*), 50—100g

Method of preparation & administration: Pound the peach seeds into a mash, add water, to obtain a dilute extract, and remove the dregs. Cook the rice in this extract into a porridge.

4
Abnormal Vaginal Discharge (*Dai Xia*)

Lotus Seed Congee
(*Lian He Zhou*)

Functions: Supplements the kidneys and secures the essence, fortifies the spleen and stops abnormal vaginal discharge

Indications: Excessive white vaginal discharge due to vacuity weakness, low back soreness, lack of strength

Ingredients: Semen Nelumbinis Nuciferae (*Lian Zi*, remove the center), Semen Euryalis Ferocis (*Qian Shi*), 100g each, fresh Folium Nelumbinis Nuciferae (*i.e.*, Lotus Leaves, *Xian He Ye*), 50g, Semen Oryzae Glutinosae (*i.e.*, Glutinous Rice, *Nuo Mi*), 50g, Granulated Sugar (*Sha Tang*), a suitable amount

Method of preparation & administration: Cook as usual into porridge. After cooking, add a little sugar to taste and eat.

Gingko Congee
(*Bai Guo Zhou*)

Functions: Warms the lungs and boosts the qi, stops cough and stabilizes panting (*i.e.*, stops asthma), stops abnormal vaginal discharge and turbidity, restrains urination

Indications: Enduring cough, qi panting (*i.e.*, asthma), white vaginal discharge, spermatorrhea, polyuria

Ingredients: Semen Gingkonis Bilobae (*Bai Guo*), 10g, Semen Oryzae Sativae (*i.e.*, Polished Rice, *Jing Mi*), 100g

Method of preparation & administration: First decoct the Gingko in water, remove the dregs, and reserve the liquid. Then cook the rice in this liquid into a porridge. Eat 3 times per day.

Powdered Poria Congee
(*Fu Ling Fen Zhou*)

Functions: Fortifies the spleen and eliminates dampness

Indications: Excessive white vaginal discharge due to spleen vacuity and dampness

Ingredients: Powdered Sclerotium Poriae Cocos (*Fu Ling Fen*), Semen Oryzae Sativae (*i.e.*, Polished Rice, *Jing Mi*), Fructus Zizyphi Jujubae (*Da Zao*), all in suitable amounts

Method of preparation & administration: Cook the above ingredients into porridge as usual and eat.

Lotus Seed, Jujube & Glutinous Rice Congee
(*Lian Zao Nuo Mi*)

Functions: Supplements the spleen and kidneys and stops abnormal vaginal discharge

Indications: Excessive white vaginal discharge due to spleen/kidney dual vacuity

Ingredients: Semen Nelumbinis Nuciferae (*Lian Zi*), 50g, Fructus Zizyphi Jujubae (*Da Zao*), 10 pieces, Semen Oryzae Glutinosae (*i.e.*, Glutinous Rice, *Nuo Mi*), 50g

Method of preparation & administration: Cook the above 3 ingredients into porridge as usual and eat 2 times per day in the morning and evening.

5
Miscarriage (*Liu Chan*)

Chicken & Glutinous Millet Congee
(*Mu Ji Huang Mi Zhou*)

Functions: Boosts the qi and nourishes the blood, quiets the fetus and calms the orientations (*i.e.*, the emotions)

Indications: Habitual miscarriage

Ingredients: Old Female Chicken (4-5 years old or older, *Lao Mu Ji*), 1 piece, Semen Setariae Glutinosae, (*i.e.*, Glutinous Millet, *Xiao Huang Mi*), 250g

Method of preparation & administration: First, kill the chicken and remove its skin and guts. Cook into soup. Then use this chicken soup to cook the glutinous millet into porridge. One may eat this as one wishes.

Chicken & Glutinous Rice Congee
(Mu Ji Nuo Mi Zhou)

Functions: Supplements vacuity, stops bleeding, quiets the fetus

Indications: Habitual miscarriage

Ingredients: Female Chicken (*Mu Ji*), 1 piece, Squid (*Mo Du Yu*), 1 large strip, Semen Oryzae Glutinosae (*i.e.*, Glutinous Rice, *Nuo Mi*), 150g, Salt (*Yan*), a small amount

Method of preparation & administration: First kill the chicken and remove the skin and guts. Then cook this and the squid into soup. Then use the soup to make porridge with the rice. Continue cooking and add some salt to taste. The chicken and squid should be cooked right in the porridge. For habitual miscarriage, eat this porridge for 2-3 whole months before conceiving and 1-2 times per month after conceiving. It is okay to eat this on a regular basis.

6
Hastening Delivery Formulas
(Cui Sheng Fang)

Sweet Potato Congee
(Yu Tou Zhou)

Functions: Scatters nodulation, loosens the intestines, and descends the qi

Indications: Dry stools, non-discharge of the lochia

Ingredients: Sweet Potato (*Yu Tou*), 250g, Semen Oryzae Sativae (*i.e.*, Polished Rice, *Da Mi*), 50g, Salt (*Yan*), a small amount

Method of preparation & administration: Remove the skin of the sweet potato, wash the rice, and make porridge out of these 2 ingredients. Eat with a little salt to flavor.

Cannabis Seed Congee
(Da Ma Zhou)

Functions: Moistens the intestines, opens strangury, quickens the blood

Indications: Postpartum blood vacuity constipation, inhibition of urination, joints congealed and astringed, wind *bi*, channel *bi*, etc.

Ingredients: Semen Cannabis Sativae (*Da Ma Ren*), 10g, Semen Oryzae Sativae (*i.e.*, Polished Rice, *Jing Mi*), 50g

Method of preparation & administration: First mash the Cannabis seed and boil in water. Afterwards add the liquid to the rice and cook into porridge. Eat 1 time each day in the morning and night.

7
Supplementing & Nourishing Formulas for Postpartum Vacuity Conditions
(Chan Hou Zhe Xu Zheng De Bu Yang Fang)

Soybean Milk & Rice Congee
(Dou Jiang Da Mi Zhou)

Functions: Regulates and harmonizes the spleen and stomach, clears heat and moistens dryness

Indications: Postpartum bodily vacuity and dryness

Ingredients: Soybean Milk (*Dou Jiang*), 2 bowls, Semen Oryzae Sativae (*i.e.*, Polished Rice, *Da Mi*), 50g, White Sugar (*Bai Tang*), a suitable amount

Method of preparation & administration: First wash the rice. Then cook the rice in the soy milk to make porridge. Add sugar to taste and eat each morning on an empty stomach.

8
Postpartum Agalactia (*Chan Hou Ru Shao*)

Aduki Bean Congee
(*Chi Xiao Dou Zhou*)

Functions: Descends the qi and opens the breasts

Indications: Postpartum scanty lactation

Ingredients: Semen Phaseoli Calcarati (*Chi Xiao Dou*), a suitable amount

Method of preparation & administration: Cook into porridge as usual and eat.

9
Acute Mastitis, Breast Abscess
(*Ji Xing Ru Xian Yan, Ru Yong*)

Dandelion Congee
(*Pu Gong Ying Zhou*)

Functions: Clears heat and resolves toxins, disperses swelling and scatters nodulation

Indications: Acute mastitis, breast abscesses, acute pharyngitis, clove sores and hot toxins, urinary tract infections, infectious hepatitis, upper respiratory tract infections

Ingredients: Fresh Herba Cum Radice Taraxaci Mongolici (*i.e.*, Dandelion, *Pu Gong Ying*), 30g, Semen Oryzae Sativae (*i.e.*, Polished Rice, *Jing Mi*), 50g, Granulated Sugar (*Bing Tang*), a suitable amount

Method of preparation & administration: First wash and chop finely the dandelion. Decoct in water, remove the dregs, and reserve 200ml of the liquid. Add this and 400ml more water to the rice and sugar and cook into porridge. Eat warm 2 times per day. Three to 5 days equal 1 course of treatment.

10
Breast Distension & Pain
(*Ru Fang Zhang Tong*)

Green (Orange) Peel Congee
(*Qing Pi Zhou*)

Functions: Courses the liver and breaks the qi, disperses accumulations and transforms stagnation

Indications: Breast swelling and pain (as in PMS), chest and lateral costal swelling and pain, *shan* qi swelling and pain

Ingredients: Pericarpium Viridis Citri Reticulatae (*Qing Pi*), 10g, Semen Oryzae Sativae (*i.e.*, Polished Rice, *Jing Mi*), 50g

Method of preparation & administration: First decoct the green orange peel in water, remove the dregs, and reserve the liquid. Add water to the rice and cook into porridge as usual. Finally, add the reserved medicinal liquid and mix thoroughly. Eat warm 2 times per day.

11
Infertility (*Bu Yun Zheng*)

Cistanches & Lamb Congee
(*Cong Rong Yang Rou Zhou*)

Functions: Supplements the kidneys and warms the uterus

Indications: Female infertility due to kidney yang vacuity

Ingredients: Herba Cistanchis (*Rou Cong Rong*), 15g, Lamb (*Yang Rou*), 100g, Semen Oryzae Sativae (*i.e.*, Polished Rice, *Jing Mi*), Herba Alli Fistulosi (*i.e.*, Scallion, *Cong*), Rhizoma Zingiberis (*i.e.*, Ginger, *Jiang*), Salt (*Yan*), each a small amount

Method of preparation & administration: First decoct the Cistanches, remove the dregs, and reserve the liquid. Then slice the lamb and put in the liquid along with the rice. Cook into porridge. Add scallions, ginger, and salt to taste.

Contraindications: Do not eat in summer.

Deer Antler Gelatin Congee (*Lu Jiao Jiao Zhou*)

Functions: Supplements the kidneys and fills the essence

Indications: Essence insufficiency infertility

Ingredients: Colla Cornu Cervi (*Lu Jiao Jiao*), 20g, Semen Oryzae Sativae (*i.e.*, Polished Rice, *Jing Mi*), 100g, fresh Rhizoma Zingiberis (*i.e.*, Fresh Ginger, *Sheng Jiang*), 3 slices

Method of preparation & administration: First cook the rice into porridge. Then add the powdered deer antler gelatin and ginger. Eat for 3-5 days, most suitably in the winter.

Amethyst Congee (*Zi Shi Ying Zhou*)

Functions: Settles the heart and quiets the spirit, warms the lungs and supplements the center, warms the uterus

Indications: Vacuity taxation palpitations, lung vacuity cough, vacuity cold of the sea of blood in women causing infertility

Ingredients: Fluoritum (*i.e.*, Amethyst, *Zi Shi Ying*), 15g, Semen Oryzae Glutinosae (*i.e.*, Glutinous Rice, *Nuo Mi*), 100g, Red Sugar (*i.e.*, Brown Sugar, *Hong Tang*), a suitable amount

Method of preparation & administration: First decoct the amethyst in 300ml of water down to 150ml. Remove the dregs and reserve the liquid. Add the rice and sugar and another 500ml of water. Cook into porridge and eat each morning and evening on an empty stomach.

CHAPTER 3

PEDIATRICS
(XIAO ER KE)

1
Pediatric Rashes & Pox
(Xiao Er Zhen Dou)

Basil Congee
(Xiang Cai Zhou)

Functions: Effuses sweat and recedes rashes, disperses food and descends the qi

Indications: The initial stage of pediatric measles

Ingredients: Herba Ocimi Basilici (*i.e.*, Basil, *Xiang Cai*), 50g, Semen Oryzae Sativae (*i.e.*, Polished Rice, *Jing Mi*), 50g, Red Sugar (*i.e.*, Brown Sugar, *Hong Tang*), a small amount

Method of preparation & administration: First cook the rice into porridge as usual. Then add the basil and bring to a boil 1 time. Add sugar to taste and eat warm.

Sesame Stalk & Glutinous Rice Congee
(Zhi Ma Gan Nuo Mi Zhou)

Functions: Scatters wind heat

Indications: Measles rashes that do not thoroughly come to the surface

Ingredients: Caulis Sesami Indici (*Zhi Ma Gan*), 12 stalks, Semen Oryzae Glutinosae (*i.e.*, Glutinous Rice, *Nuo Mi*), 200g

Method of preparation & administration: First cut the stalks into pieces and boil in 2,000ml of water. Afterwards, filter out this water and use to cook the glutinous rice into porridge. Divide into 2 portions and take. Typically, one will heal after using this formula 3 times.

Beet Congee
(*Tian Cai Zhou*)

Functions: Clears heat and recedes rashes, fortifies the spleen and boosts the stomach

Indications: Measles rashes that do not thoroughly come to the surface

Ingredients: Fresh Beets (*Xin Xian Tian Cai*), 200g, Semen Oryzae Sativae (*i.e.*, Polished Rice, *Jing Mi*), 100g

Method of preparation & administration: First wash the beets and cut them into pieces. Cook the rice and beets into porridge as usual and eat warm 2 times per day.

2
Pediatric Night Sweats
(*Xiao Er Dao Han*)

Wheat & Glutinous Rice Congee
(*Xiao Mai Nuo Mi Zhou*)

Functions: Strengthens and fortifies the spleen and stomach, restrains sweat and calms the spirit

Indications: Spleen vacuity in the aftermath of disease, night sweats, spontaneous sweating, and other such conditions

Ingredients: Fructus Tritici (*i.e.*, Wheat, *Xiao Mai*), 60g, Semen Oryzae Glutinosae (*i.e.*, Glutinous Rice, *Nuo Mi*), 30g, Fructus

Zizyphi Jujubae (*Da Zao*), 15 pieces, White Sugar (*Bai Tang*), a small amount

Method of preparation & administration: Cook the first 3 ingredients into porridge as usual. Then add sugar to taste. Eat 2 times per day.

3
Pediatric Bedwetting
(*Xiao Er Yi Niao*)

Female Chicken Congee
(*Mu Ji Zhou*)

Functions: Supplements the kidneys and boosts the qi

Indications: Pediatric enuresis

Ingredients: Yellow Female Chicken (*Mu Huang Ji*), 1, Semen Oryzae Sativae (*i.e.*, Polished Rice, *Jing Mi*), 120g, Radix Astragali Membranacei (*Huang Qi*), 30g, prepared Radix Rehmanniae (*Shu Di*), 15g

Method of preparation & administration: Skin and gut the chicken and boil with the Astragalus and Rehmannia until thoroughly cooked. Remove the medicinals and chicken, add the rice, and cook into porridge.

4
Pediatric Malnutrition
(*Xiao Er Gan Ji*)

Chicken Gizzard Powder Congee
(*Ji Zhun Fen Zhou*)

Functions: Disperses accumulations and transforms food
Indications: Food stagnation pediatric *gan*

Ingredients: Endothelium Corneum Gigeriae Galli (*Ji Nei Jin*), 6 pieces, Pericarpium Citri Reticulatae (*Chen Pi*), 3g, Fructus Amomi (*Sha Ren*), 1.5g, Semen Oryzae Sativae (*i.e.*, Polished Rice, *Jing Mi*), 30g, White Sugar (*Bai Tang*), a suitable amount

Method of preparation & administration: Grind the chicken gizzards, orange peel, and Amomum into a fine powder. Cook the rice and water into porridge and add the powder when the porridge is done, cooking for a few minutes more.

5
Hundred Day Cough (*i.e.*, Whooping Cough) (*Bai Ri Ke*)

Bamboo Juice Congee (*Zhu Li Zhou*)

Functions: Clears heat and transforms phlegm

Indications: Pediatric whooping cough due to phlegm heat

Ingredients: Succus Bambusae (*Zhu Li*), Semen Setariae Italicae (*i.e.*, Millet, *Su Mi*), equal parts

Method of preparation & administration: Cook the millet into porridge with water and then add the bamboo juice. Mix thoroughly and eat.

Kumquat Congee (*Jin Ju Zhou*)

Functions: Stops cough and transforms phlegm, harmonizes the center and stops pain

Indications: Pediatric whooping cough, cough, phlegm, and panting (*i.e.*, asthma) in the elderly, wind cold common cold causing cough, indigestion, stomach and abdominal distention and pain, *shan* qi aching and pain, diminished appetite due to common cold in any of the four seasons

Ingredients: Fresh Kumquat (*Xian Jin Ju*), 5 pieces, Semen Oryzae Sativae (*i.e.*, Polished Rice, *Da Mi*), 30g

Method of preparation & administration: First cook the rice into porridge as usual. Then add the kumquats and a small amount of sugar and eat.

6
Pediatric Diarrhea (*Xiao Er Fu Xie*)

Three Grains Congee
(*San Mi Zhou*)

Functions: Fortifies the spleen and harmonizes the stomach

Indications: Pediatric diarrhea due to spleen qi vacuity

Ingredients: Semen Sorghi Vulgaris (*i.e.*, Husked Sorghum, *Gao Liang Mi*), 50g, Semen Oryzae Sativae (*i.e.*, Polished Rice, *Jing Mi*), 50g, Semen Panici Miliacei (*i.e.*, Broomcorn Millet, *Shu Mi*), 50g, Cera Flava (*i.e.*, Beeswax, *Feng La*), 6g

Method of preparation & administration: First cook the sorghum in water till it has boiled 3 times. Remove the dregs and reserve the liquid. Cook the rice in this liquid till it has boiled 3 times. Remove the dregs and reserve the liquid. Then cook the broomcorn millet in this liquid till it has boiled 3 times. Remove the dregs and press out any remaining liquid from the millet. Add the wax while hot to this liquid and allow to melt. Administer 10ml each time, 2 times a day in the morning and evening.

7
Pediatric Mumps
(*Xiao Er Sa Xian Yan*)

Mung Bean & Cabbage Heart Congee
(*Lu Dou Cai Xin Zhou*)

Functions: Clears and resolves hot toxins, eliminates vexation and stops thirst

Indications: Pediatric mumps

Ingredients: Semen Phaseoli Munginis (*i.e.*, Mung Beans, *Lu Dou*), 100g, Cabbage Hearts (*Cai Xin*), 3 whole ones

Method of preparation & administration: First cook the mung beans into porridge as usual. Then add the white cabbage hearts and cook till done. Divide into 2 portions and eat 2 times each day for 4 days continuously.

CHAPTER *4*

THE FIVE OFFICIALS
(*I.E., EARS, EYES, NOSE, LIPS & TONGUE*)
(*WU GUAN KE*)

1
Blurred Vision (*Hua Yan*)

Chicken Livers & Rice Congee
(*Ji Gan Da Mi Zhou*)

Functions: Supplements the liver and nourishes the blood, brightens the eyes

Indications: Blurred vision, night blindness, dimming of vision in the elderly

Ingredients: Chicken Livers (*Ji Gan*), 2, Semen Oryzae Sativae (*i.e.*, Polished Rice, *Da Mi*), 100g, Salt (*Yan*), a small amount

Method of preparation & administration: Make into porridge as usual and eat morning and night.

Sheep Liver Congee
(*Yang Gan Zhou*)

Functions: Supplements the liver and brightens the eyes

Indications: Night blindness, blurred vision, pediatric *gan* eyes

Ingredients: Sheep Liver (*Yang Gan*), 60g, Semen Oryzae Sativae (*i.e.*, Polished Rice, *Da Mi*), 100g, Herba Alli Fistulosi (*i.e.*, Fresh Scallion, *Sheng Cong*), 3 stalks

Method of preparation & administration: First remove any membranes from the liver and cut into pieces. Also chop the scallions. Then boil in water. Add the rice and cook into porridge. Eat daily.

Sweet Potato Congee
(*Hong Shu Zhou*)

Functions: Fortifies the spleen and boosts the stomach, boosts the qi and warms the center

Indications: Night blindness, vitamin A deficiency, stagnant blood in the stools, constipation, damp heat jaundice, etc.

Ingredients: Fresh Sweet Potato (*Xin Xian Hong Shu*), 250g, Semen Oryzae Sativae (*i.e.*, Polished Rice, *Jing Mi*), 200g, White Sugar (*Bai Tang*), a suitable amount

Method of preparation & administration: Cook into porridge as usual, add sugar to taste, and eat warm morning and evening. However, do not overeat. Prolonged consumption of sweet flavored foods leads to stomach disease.

Lycium Berries Congee
(*Qi Zi Zhou*)

Functions: Supplements the liver and kidneys and brightens the eyes

Indications: Liver/kidney yin vacuity, dizziness and vertigo, diminished visual acuity, low back and knee soreness and weakness, impotence, spermatorrhea, diabetes mellitus, high blood pressure, chronic hepatitis, arteriosclerosis

Ingredients: Fructus Lycii Chinensis (*Gou Qi Zi*), 20g, Semen Oryzae Glutinosae (*i.e.*, Glutinous Rice, *Nuo Mi*), 50g, White Sugar (*Bai Tang*), a small amount

Method of preparation & administration: Add water and cook into porridge as usual. Eat warm every day in the morning and evening. It is ok to eat this over a prolonged period of time.

2
Senile Cataracts
(*Lao Nian Xiang Bai Nei Zhang*)

Liver & Spleen Dual Supplementing Congee
(*Gan Pi Shuang Bu Zhou*)

Functions: Supplements the spleen, liver, and kidneys

Indications: Spleen qi vacuity and liver blood vacuity senile cataracts

Ingredients: Excrementum Vespertilii (*Ye Ming Sha*), 9g, Radix Dioscoreae Oppositae (*Shan Yao*), 30g, Semen Cuscutae (*Tu Si Zi*), 9g, Semen Oryzae Sativae (*i.e.*, Polished Rice, *Jing Mi*), 60g, Red Sugar (*i.e.*, Brown Sugar, *Hong Tang*), a suitable amount

Method of preparation & administration: Wrap the bat feces, Chinese yam, and Cuscuta in a cloth bag. Decoct in 2,500ml of water down to 1,500ml. Use the resulting liquid to make porridge from the rice and brown sugar. Take 2 times per day for 15-20 days continuously.

3
Conjunctivitis (*Yan Chi Zhong Tong*)

Two Creating Brightness Congee
(*Shuan Jue Ming Zhou*)

Functions: Nourishes the liver and represses yang, clears heat from the liver and brightens the eyes

Indications: Conjunctivitis, photophobia, head distention and pain, dizziness, blurred vision, dry, astringent eyes, and other such symptoms of liver/kidney yin vacuity and liver yang hyperactivity

Ingredients: Concha Haliotidis (*Shi Jue Ming*), 25g, Semen Cassiae Torae (*Jue Ming Zi*), 10g, Flos Chrysanthemi Morifolii (*Ju Hua*), 15g, Semen Oryzae Sativae (*i.e.*, Polished Rice, *Jing Mi*), 100g, Granulated Sugar (*Bing Tang*), 6g

Method of preparation & administration: First stir-fry the Cassia seeds until they become fragrant. Decoct the Chrysanthemum flowers, Cassia seeds, and abalone shell, remove the dregs, and reserve the liquid. Cook the rice into congee with water and this reserved liquid. Add the sugar and eat 2 times per day in the morning and evening. Three to 5 days equal 1 course of treatment.

4
Tinnitus (*Er Ming*)

Chrysanthemum Congee
(*Ju Hua Zhou*)

Functions: Clears the liver, brightens the eyes and ears

Indications: Tinnitus due to hyperactive liver yang

Ingredients: Flos Chrysanthemi Morifolii (*Ju Hua*), 15g, Semen Oryzae Sativae (*i.e.*, Polished Rice, *Jing Mi*), 60g

Method of preparation & administration: Powder the Chrysanthemum and make porridge with it and the rice as usual. Take 1 time per day for several days continuously.

Magnetite Congee
(*Ci Shi Zhou*)

Functions: Supplements the kidneys, quiets the spirit and orientation, improves the hearing, and brightens the eyes

Indications: Deafness, tinnitus, dizziness, vertigo, heart palpitations, and insomnia in the elderly due to kidney vacuity

Ingredients: Magnetitum (*Ci Shi*), 60g, Pork Kidneys (*Zhu Yao Zi*), 1 pair, Semen Oryzae Sativae (*i.e.*, Polished Rice, *Da Mi*), 100g

Method of preparation & administration: First pound and powder the Magnetite and decoct in 200-300ml of water for 1 hour. Remove the dregs and reserve the liquid. Cut up the pork kidneys and remove the membranes. Add the medicinal liquid and 800ml of water to the rice and kidneys and cook into porridge. Eat warm each evening before going to bed.

Acorus Congee
(*Chang Pu Zhou*)

Functions: Aromatically and fragrantly transforms dampness, opens the portals, and stabilizes the spirit

Indications: Tinnitus, deafness, mania and withdrawal, poor memory, fetal leakage, *yong* swellings

Ingredients: Rhizoma Acori Graminei (*Shi Chang Pu*), 5g, Semen Oryzae Sativae (*i.e.*, Polished Rice, *Jing Mi*), 50g, Granulated Sugar (*Bing Tang*), a suitable amount

Method of preparation & administration: Grind the Acorus into powder. Then cook the rice and the sugar into porridge using approximately 450ml of water. Stir in the Acorus powder and continue cooking for a short time longer. Eat warm 2 times per day.

5
Pharyngitis (*Yan Yan*)

Relieve the Exterior & Disinhibit the Throat Congee
(*Jie Biao Li Yan Zhou*)

Functions: Relieves the exterior and disinhibits the throat

Indications: Wind heat sore throat

Ingredients: Spica Seu Flos Schizonepetae Tenuifoliae (*Jing Jie Sui*), 9g, Radix Platycodi Grandiflori (*Jie Geng*), 12g, Radix Glycyrrhizae (*Gan Cao*), 6g, Semen Oryzae Sativae (*i.e.*, Polished Rice, *Jing Mi*), 60g

Method of preparation & administration: Wrap the first 3 ingredients in a cloth bag and decoct. Remove the dregs and reserve the liquid. Cook the rice in this liquid into a porridge. Eat 1 time per day for several days continuously.

6
Tonsillitis (*Pian Tao Ti Yan*)

Dandelion Congee
(*Pu Gong Ying Zhou*)

Functions: Clears heat and resolves toxins

Indications: Acute tonsillitis

Ingredients: Herba Cum Radice Taraxaci Mongolici (*Pu Gong Ying*), 60g, Semen Oryzae Sativae (*i.e.*, Polished Rice, *Jing Mi*), 100g

Method of preparation & administration: Decoct the dandelion in water, remove the dregs, and reserve the liquid. Cook the rice in this liquid to make porridge. Eat warm 2-3 times per day. Three to 5 days equals 1 course of treatment.

7
Disease of the Voice (*Sang Yin Bing*)

Pear Juice Congee
(*Li Zhi Zhou*)

Functions: Supplements the lungs and moistens dryness

Indications: Hoarseness due to overuse, as in singers and speakers

Ingredients: Pear (*Li*), 3-5 whole ones, Semen Oryzae Sativae (*i.e.*, Polished Rice, *Jing Mi*), 50g, Granulated Sugar (*Bing Tang*), a suitable amount

Method of preparation & administration: Wash 3-5 pears and cut into pieces. Pound and strain to juice. Cook the resulting juice with the rice and granulated sugar in 400ml of water into a porridge. Take slightly warm 2-3 times per day.

CHAPTER 5

DERMATOLOGY
(PI FU KE)

1
Facial Beautification Formula
(Mei Rong Yan Zhe Fang)

**Coix Congee
(Yi Mi Zhou)**

Functions: Fortifies the spleen, disinhibits dampness, clears heat

Indications: Pimples during puberty

Ingredients: Semen Coicis Lachryma-jobi (*Yi Yi Mi*), 50g, White Sugar (*Bai Tang*), 15g

Method of preparation & administration: Wash the Coix, add water, and cook into porridge. Stir in the sugar and eat 1 time per day continuously for 1 month.

2
Yellow Water Sores
(*i.e.*, all sorts of blistery, suppurative lesions)
(*Huang Shui Chuang*)

Purslane Congee
(*Ma Chi Xian Zhou*)

Functions: Clears heat and resolves toxins

Indications: All types of pustular, suppurative skin lesions and sores

Ingredients: Herba Portulacae Oleraceae (*i.e.*, Purslane, *Ma Chi Xian*), 30g, Semen Oryzae Sativae (*i.e.*, Polished Rice, *Jing Mi*), 50g

Method of preparation & administration: Cook into porridge as usual and eat.

Burdock Root Congee
(*Niu Bang Zhou*)

Functions: Clears heat and resolves toxins

Indications: All types of pustular, suppurative skin lesions and sores

Ingredients: Succus Radicis Arctii Lappae (*i.e.*, Burdock Root Juice, *Niu Bang Gen Zhi*), 50g, Semen Oryzae Sativae (*i.e.*, Polished Rice, *Jing Mi*), 60g

Method of preparation & administration: Crush and press of 50ml of juice from a suitable amount of fresh burdock root. Add to the rice and water and cook into porridge.

Mung Bean & Wheat Congee
(*Lu Mai Zhou*)

Functions: Clears heat, resolves toxins

Indications: Sores, ulcers, toxic swellings, toxins from alcohol and foods

Ingredients: Semen Phaseoli Munginis (*i.e.*, M ung Beans, *Lu Dou*), 30g, Semen Oryzae Glutinosae (*i.e.*, Glutinous Rice, *Nuo Mi*), 30g, Semen Tritici (*i.e.*, Wheat, *Xiao Mai*), 30g

Method of preparation & administration: First stir-fry the above 3 ingredients. Then grind them into powder and store for use. Each time, use 30g and cook in boiling water into porridge.

Agrimonia & Glutinous Rice Congee
(*Xian He Nuo Mi Zhou*)

Functions: Moves the blood, disperses swelling

Indications: Pussy swellings, toxic swellings

Ingredients: Fresh Radix Agrimoniae Pilosae (*Xian Xian He Cao Gen*), 250g, Semen Oryzae Glutinosae (*i.e.*, Glutinous Rice, *Nuo Mi*), a suitable amount

Method of preparation & administration: First wash the Agrimonia. Then put it and the rice in water and cook into porridge. While the porridge is still hot, remove the Agrimonia and add a little sugar to taste before eating. Take 1 time per day for 3-5 days continuously.

CHAPTER 6

LIFE-LENGTHENING TO 100 YEARS, ENRICHING & SUPPLEMENTING FORMULAS
(CHANG MING BAI NIAN DE ZI BU FANG)

1
Yin-supplementing Formulas
(Bu Yin Fang)

Butter & Honey Congee
(Su Mi Zhou)

Functions: Nourishes the five viscera, supplements the qi and blood, makes the skin moist and glossy

Indications: Vacuity of the five viscera, bodily debility and weakness, vacuity taxation fever, lung vacuity enduring cough with phlegm containing blood, constipation due to intestinal dryness, rough skin, withered hair, etc.

Ingredients: Butter (*Su You*), 30g, Honey (*Mi Tang*), 15g, Semen Oryzae Sativae (*i.e.*, Polished Rice, *Jing Mi*), 60g

Method of preparation & administration: Cook the rice, butter, and honey into porridge and eat hot, 2 times per day, morning and evening.

Prepared Rehmannia Congee
(*Shu Di Zhou*)

Functions: Supplements kidney yin and nourishes liver blood

Indications: Blood vacuity sallow, yellowish complexion, dizziness, heart palpitations, steaming bone and tidal fever, night sweats, spermatorrhea, low back and knee soreness and weakness, menstrual irregularity, and wasting and thirsting

Ingredients: Prepared Radix Rehmanniae (*Shu Di*), 30g, Semen Oryzae Sativae (*i.e.*, Polished Rice, *Jing Mi*), 40g

Method of preparation & administration: First decoct the Rehmannia in 500ml of water, remove the dregs, and reserve the liquid. Add this liquid to the rice and more water if necessary and cook into porridge. Eat warm 1 time per day on an empty stomach. Ten days equal 1 course of treatment.

Achyranthes Congee
(*Niu Xi Zhou*)

Functions: Clears heat and eliminates vexation

Indications: The sequelae of febrile diseases, vacuity taxation, emaciation, vexatious aching of the four limbs, dry mouth, strong fever

Ingredients: Tender, new Folium Achyranthis Bidentatae (*Niu Xi Miao Ye*), Folium Solani Nigri (*Long Gui Ye*), Radix Rehmanniae (*Sheng Di Huang*), 10g each, Semen Oryzae Sativae (*i.e.*, Polished Rice, *Jing Mi*), 100g

Method of preparation & administration: First decoct the first 3 medicinals, remove the dregs, and reserve the liquid. Use this liquid to make porridge out of the rice. Eat on an empty stomach.

Dendrobium Congee
(*Shi Hu Zhou*)

Functions: Nourishes the stomach and engenders fluids, nourishes yin and clears heat

Indications: Damaged fluids due to a febrile disease, heart vexation, oral thirst, unhealthy yin vacuity, stomach vacuity cramping pain, dry heaves, a scant tongue coating

Ingredients: Herba Dendrobii (*Shi Hu*), 15g, Semen Oryzae Sativae (*i.e.*, Polished Rice, *Da Mi*), 50g, Granulated Sugar (*Bing Tang*), a suitable amount

Method of preparation & administration: First decoct the Dendrobium in water, remove the dregs, and reserve 100ml of liquid. Add this and more water to the rice and sugar and cook into porridge. Eat warm 2 times per day.

Mulberry Congee
(*Sang Shen Zhou*)

Functions: Supplements the liver and boosts the kidneys, enriches yin and supplements the blood, moistens the intestines, and brightens the eyes

Indications: Yin and blood insufficiency, dizziness, vertigo, insomnia, tinnitus, diminished visual acuity, premature greying of the hair, blood vacuity constipation, neurasthenia, anemia, yin vacuity high blood pressure, etc.

Ingredients: Fresh Fructus Mori Albi (*i.e.*, Mulberries, *Sang Shen*), 30g (or dry, 20g), Semen Oryzae Glutinosae (*i.e.*, Glutinous Rice, *Nuo Mi*), 50g, Granulated Sugar (*Bing Tang*), a suitable amount

Method of preparation & administration: Cook into porridge in 400ml of water. Eat warm each morning on an empty stomach.

2
Yang-supplementing Formulas
(*Bu Yang Fang*)

Chinese Chive Congee
(*Jiu Cai Zhou*)

Functions: Supplements the kidneys and invigorates yang, fortifies the spleen and warms the stomach

Indications: Chilly pain in the abdomen, loose stool or constipation, enduring dysentery due to vacuity cold, impotence, premature ejaculation, spermatorrhea, polyuria, urinary incontinence, abnormal vaginal discharge, low back and knee soreness and weakness, dysmenorrhea, metrorrhagia, and other such conditions due to kidney/spleen yang vacuity

Ingredients: Herba Allii Tuberosi (*i.e.*, Chinese Chives, *Jiu Cai*), 60g, Semen Oryzae Sativae (*i.e.*, Polished Rice, *Jing Mi*), 60g, Salt (*Yan*), a small amount

Method of preparation & administration: Cut the chives into small pieces. Make the rice into porridge as usual and put in the chives. Salt to taste and continue cooking a few minutes more. Eat 2 times per day in the morning and evening.

Cistanches & Lamb Congee
(*Cong Rong Yang Rou Zhou*)

Functions: Supplements the kidneys and invigorates yang, fortifies the spleen and frees the stool

Indications: Kidney yang vacuity impotence, spermatorrhea, premature ejaculation, infertility in women, chilly pain in the low back and knees, polyuria, nocturia, bodily vacuity weakness, internal damage due to overtaxation, aversion to cold, cold limbs, constipation due to insufficiency of yang in the elderly

Ingredients: Herba Cistanchis (*Rou Cong Rong*), 15g, Lamb (*Yang Rou*), 60g, Semen Oryzae Sativae (*i.e.*, Polished Rice, *Jing Mi*), 60g, Salt (*Yan*), a small amount, Bulbus Allii Fistulosi (*i.e.*, Scallions, *Cong Bai*), 2 pieces, fresh Rhizoma Zingiberis (*i.e.*, Fresh Ginger, *Sheng Jiang*), 3 slices

Method of preparation & administration: First decoct the Cistanches, remove the dregs, and reserve the liquid. Use this liquid to make porridge from the rice and lamb. Add salt, scallions, and ginger to taste. Eat 2 times per day in the morning and evening.

Sparrow Medicinal Congee
(Que Er Yao Zhou)

Functions: Strengthens yang qi, supplements essence and blood, boosts the liver and kidneys

Indications: Kidney qi insufficiency causing impotence, spermatorrhea, daybreak diarrhea, dizziness, blurred vision, unclear speech, deafness, tinnitus, urinary incontinence, abnormal vaginal discharge, etc.

Ingredients: Passer Montanus Saturatus (*i.e.*, Sparrow, *Que Er*), 5 whole ones, Semen Cuscutae (*Tu Si Zi*), 45g, Fructus Rubi (*Fu Pen Zi*), 15g, Fructus Lycii Chinensis (*Gou Qi Zi*), 30g, Semen Oryzae Sativae (*Jing Mi*), 60g, Salt (*Yan*), a small amount, Bulbus Allii Fistulosi (*i.e.*, Scallion), 2 stalks, fresh Rhizoma Zingiberis (*i.e.*, fresh Ginger, *Sheng Jiang*), 3 slices

Method of preparation & administration: First decoct the Cuscuta, Rubus, and Lycium, remove the dregs, and reserve the liquid. Skin and gut the sparrows, wash and stir-fry in wine. Then cook the rice, sparrows, and medicinal decoction with a suitable amount of water to make porridge. Just before it is finished, add salt, scallions, and ginger and continue cooking a few minutes more. Eat 2 times per day on an empty stomach, once in the morning and once in the evening. Three to 5 days equal 1 course of treatment.

Contraindications: Those with hyperactive sex drive or fever should not use this congee. It should also only be eaten in the winter.

3
Qi-supplementing Formulas (*Bu Qi Fang*)

Ginseng Congee
(*Ren Shen Zhou*)

Functions: Boosts the original qi and vitalizes the essence spirit, supplements the spleen, lung, and heart qi

Indications: Spleen vacuity symptoms such as emaciation due to prolonged disease, lack of appetite, and loose stools, lack of strength, fatigued spirit, and physical exhaustion; lung vacuity symptoms such as shortness of the breath and vacuity panting (*i.e.*, asthma); and heart vacuity symptoms such as palpitations, insomnia, and poor memory

Ingredients: Powdered Radix Panacis Ginseng (*Ren Shen Fen*), 3g, Semen Oryzae Sativae (*i.e.*, Polished Rice, *Jing Mi*), 100g, Granulated Sugar (*Bing Tang*), a suitable amount

Method of preparation & administration: Cook the powdered Ginseng into porridge with the rice and add the sugar at the end. Eat on a regular basis.

Ginseng & Poria Congee
(*Shen Ling Zhou*)

Functions: Fortifies the spleen and boosts the qi

Indications: Qi vacuity, bodily weakness, fatigue, pale facial color, poor appetite, loose stool, and other such symptoms

Ingredients: Radix Panacis Ginseng (*Ren Shen*), 5g, Sclerotium Poriae Cocos (*Fu Ling*), 20g, fresh Rhizoma Zingiberis (*i.e.*, Fresh Ginger, *Sheng Jiang*), 5g, Semen Oryzae Sativae (*i.e.*, Polished Rice, *Jing Mi*), 60g

Method of preparation & administration: Cut the Ginseng into thin slices and pound the Poria into pieces. Soak these 2 ingredients for 1/2 hour. Then decoct them in water for 30 minutes. Pour off the liquid, reserve, and decoct again. Again pour off the liquid and add to the first decoction. Add this liquid to the rice and cook into porridge as usual.

Ginseng & Chicken Congee
(*Ren Shen Ji Zhou*)

Functions: Enriches and supplements the five viscera, strengthens the body, supplements and boosts the qi and blood

Indications: Bodily vacuity and weakness in the elderly or those with chronic disease

Ingredients: Radix Panacis Ginseng (*Ren Shen*), 3g, Radix Dioscoreae Oppositae (*Shan Yao*), 6g, Semen Oryzae Sativae (*i.e.*, Polished Rice, *Da Mi*), 50g, Chicken (*Ji*), 1 whole one, Chicken Livers (*Ji Gan*), 150g

Method of preparation & administration: First cook the chicken and chicken livers in 15 bowlsful of water into soup. Slice the Ginseng, Chinese yam, and the chicken soup to the rice and cook into porridge. Add salt to taste and eat.

Codonopsis Congee
(*Dang Shen Zhou*)

Functions: Supplements the middle and boosts the qi

Indications: Qi vacuity and insufficiency, chronic cough, poor appetite, abdominal distention, loose stools, and other such spleen/lung qi vacuity conditions

Ingredients: Radix Codonopsis Pilosulae (*Dang Shen*), 30g, Semen Oryzae Sativae (*i.e.*, Polished Rice, *Da Mi*), 50g, White Sugar (*Bai Tang*), a small amount

Method of preparation & administration: Cook the rice and Codonopsis in water into porridge as usual and add the sugar at the end to taste. Eat warm.

Pseudostellaria Congee
(*Tai Zi Shen Zhou*)

Functions: Supplements the qi and engenders fluids

Indications: Bodily vacuity in the aftermath of disease, yin vacuity/lung dryness chronic cough with scant phlegm, insomnia, excessive dreams

Ingredients: Radix Pseudostellariae Heterophyllae (*Tai Zi Shen*), 50g, Semen Oryzae Sativae (*i.e.*, Polished Rice, *Da Mi*), 50g

Method of preparation & administration: First decoct the Pseudostellaria, remove the dregs, and reserve the liquid. Add this to the rice and cook into porridge. Eat warm in the morning and evening.

Astragalus Congee
(*Huang Qi Zhou*)

Functions: Strengthens and boosts the qi and fortifies the spleen

Indications: Qi vacuity bodily weakness, fatigue, lack of strength, diminished appetite, loose stools, anal prolapse, spontaneous sweating, night sweats, superficial edema of the face and eyes, inhibited urination, shortness of breath, heart palpitations, etc.

Ingredients: Radix Astragali Membranacei (*Huang Qi*), 20g, Semen Oryzae Sativae (*i.e.*, Polished Rice, *Jing Mi*), 50g

Method of preparation & administration: Add the Astragalus to 200ml of water and decoct down to 100ml. Remove the dregs and reserve the liquid. Add this to the rice plus another 300ml of water and cook into porridge. Eat warm in the morning and evening. Seven to 10 days equal 1 course of treatment. It is ok to add a little Red Sugar (*i.e.*, Brown Sugar, *Hong Tang*) to taste.

Supplement Righteous Qi Vacuity Congee (*Bu Xu Zheng Qi Zhou*)

Functions: Supplements the righteous qi

Indications: Vacuity detriment, taxation fatigue internal damage, vacuity debility of the five viscera, bodily weakness in the elderly, emaciation due to prolonged disease, heart palpitations, shortness of breath, spontaneous sweating, chronic diarrhea, devitalized appetite, qi vacuity superficial edema, etc.

Ingredients: Radix Astragali Membranacei (*Huang Qi*), 60g, Radix Panacis Ginseng (*Ren Shen*), 10g, Semen Oryzae Sativae (*i.e.*, Polished Rice, *Jing Mi*), 90g, White Sugar (*Bai Tang*), a small amount

Method of preparation & administration: First slowly decoct the Astragalus and Ginseng 2 times, then remove the dregs, and reserve the liquid. Divide this liquid into 2 portions. Each day, use 1 portion to cook the rice into porridge. Add a little sugar to taste after cooking. Eat each morning and evening on an empty stomach. Five days equal 1 course of treatment.

Contraindications: Do not use this congee if one is suffering from a hot pathocondition. Do not eat radishes or drink tea while taking this congee.

Atractylodes & Pork Tripe Congee (*Bai Zhu Zhu Du Zhou*)

Functions: Supplements the middle and boosts the qi, fortifies the spleen and harmonizes the stomach

Indications: Spleen qi vacuity, fatigue, shortness of breath, loose stool, poor appetite, indigestion, abdominal distention, and other such symptoms

Ingredients: Rhizoma Atractylodis Macrocephalae (*Bai Zhu*), 30g, Semen Arecae Catechu (*Bing Lang*), 10g, Pork Tripe (*Zhu Du*), 1 piece, fresh Rhizoma Zingiberis (*Sheng Jiang*), a small amount, Semen Oryzae Sativae (*i.e.*, Polished Rice, *Jing Mi*), 60g

Method of preparation & administration: Cut the pork tripe into small pieces and decoct together with the Atractylodes, Areca, and ginger. Remove the dregs and reserve the liquid. Use this liquid to cook the rice into porridge. Take 2 times per day in the morning and evening. Eat the trip with sesame oil (*Xiang You*) and soy sauce (*Jiang You*). Eat for 3-5 days. Wait for 3 days, and take again. Stop taking as soon as the symptoms are relieved.

4
Blood-supplementing Formulas
(*Bu Xue Fang*)

Barley Congee
(*Da Mai Zhou*)

Functions: Nourishes the blood and constructs the body

Indications: Prolonged eating strengthens the physical body, prevents the hair from turning white, loosens the stomach and stops distention

Ingredients: Fructus Hordei Vulgaris (*i.e.*, Barley, *Da Mai*), 100g

Method of preparation & administration: Make into porridge as usual and eat 2 times per day.

Sweet Soy Milk Congee
(*Gan Jiang Zhou*)

Functions: Supplements vacuity, stops cough, and moistens the intestines

Indications: Bodily vacuity, emaciation, enduring cough, dry stools, etc.

Ingredients: Fresh Soybean Milk (*Xian Dou Jiang*), 500ml, Semen Oryzae Sativae (*i.e.*, Polished Rice, *Da Mi*), 50g, White Sugar (*Bai Tang*), a small amount

Method of preparation & administration: First cook the rice in the soy milk and make into porridge. Then stir in the sugar to taste. Eat each morning and evening.

Black Sesame Congee
(*Hei Zhi Ma Zhou*)

Functions: Supplements the liver and kidneys, moistens the five viscera

Indications: Bodily debility in the elderly, dizziness and vertigo, emaciation, dry stools, premature greying of the hair, postpartum scanty lactation

Ingredients: Black Semen Sesami Indici (*i.e.*, Black Sesame Seeds, *Hei Zhi Ma*), 25g, Semen Oryzae Sativae (*i.e.*, Polished Rice, *Da Mi*), 50g

Method of preparation & administration: First grind the sesame seeds. Then wash the rice. Next, make into porridge as usual and eat.

Glutinous Rice & Donkey Skin Glue Congee
(Nuo Mi E Jiao Zhou)

Functions: Nourishes the blood and stops bleeding, enriches yin and moistens the lungs

Indications: Stirring of restless fetus, fetal leakage precipitating blood, blood vacuity, a sallow, yellowish facial color, dizziness and vertigo, heart palpitations, vacuity taxation hemoptysis, hematemesis, hematuria, hemafecia, etc.

Ingredients: Gelatinum Corii Asini (*E Jiao*), 20g, Semen Oryzae Glutinosae (*i.e.*, Glutinous Rice, *Nuo Mi*), 100g

Method of preparation & administration: First cook the rice into porridge. Then grind the donkey skin glue. Add it to the porridge to dissolve. Eat on an empty stomach.

Spinach Congee
(Bo Cai Zhou)

Functions: Nourishes the blood and moistens dryness

Indications: Anemia, constipation, high blood pressure

Ingredients: Spinach (*Bo Cai*), 250g, Semen Oryzae Sativae (*i.e.*, Polished Rice, *Jing Mi*), 100g, Salt (*Yan*), a suitable amount

Method of preparation & administration: Wash the spinach and cut into small pieces. Cook with the rice in water to make porridge. Eat on a regular basis.

Note: A similar blood-nourishing congee can be made from beet tops, Swiss chard, kale, collards, or other such greens.

GENERAL INDEX

A

abdomen, cramping, aching, and pain of the stomach and 80
abdominal chilly pain 77, 79, 80, 120, 145
abdominal cramping pain 71
abdominal distention 10, 48, 70, 72, 104, 109, 118, 121-123, 129, 161, 181, 184
abdominal distention and pain 48, 161
abdominal pain 121, 125, 129, 146
abdominal pain, stasis and stagnation 146
abdominal water distention and fullness 112
accumulations and stagnation 70
amebic dysentery 126
amenorrhea 143, 146, 148
anal itching 26
anal prolapse 123, 182
anemia 68, 87-89, 129, 177, 186
anemia, liver blood/kidney yin vacuity 88
anemia, spleen and heart dual vacuity 89
angina pectoris 93, 94
aphasia 98, 99
aphasia and indistinct speech 99
appetite, devitalized 48, 81, 116, 121, 128, 183
appetite, diminished 71, 75, 161, 182
appetite, scant 62
appetite, stomach vacuity lack of 88
arteriosclerosis 91, 93, 164
arthritis, rheumatic 110
ascites due to cirrhosis 107
asthma 12, 51, 53, 54, 56, 58, 64-67, 149, 161, 180
atony 12, 58, 138

B

bladder infections 37
bleeding, digestive tract 82
bleeding hemorrhoids 124
bleeding, lower burner 124
blindness, night 163, 164
blood fat, reduces 91, 92
blood pressure, chronic low 97, 98

blood pressure, high 37, 57, 89-92, 111, 114, 126, 164, 177, 186
blood vacuity 118, 138, 143, 147, 152, 165, 176, 177, 186
bloody dysentery 72, 124
bodily debility 175, 185
bodily fatigue 48
bodily vacuity weakness 62, 67, 99, 129, 152, 178, 181, 182, 185
bodily weakness 10, 58, 67, 74, 101, 180, 182, 183
bone break 103
bone break, swelling, and pain 103
bowel movements not crisp 109
brain, distended 49
breast abscess 141, 153
breast swelling and pain 154
breath, bad 48, 72
breathing, lung vacuity hurried 66
bronchitis 51-54, 60-63, 66, 75
bronchitis, acute 53
bronchitis, chronic 51, 53, 60, 75
bronchitis, pediatric 54

C

cancer, prevention of 93
cataracts, senile 165
channel *bi* 152
cheeks, flushed in the evening 85
chest and diaphragm fullness and oppression 51
chest and lateral costal aching and pain 146
chest fullness with excessive phlegm 66
chest oppression 48, 71
chest pain 93, 94
chill, fear of 43
cholecystitis 126
cholesterol, high 3, 37, 90, 91, 111
chronic diseases and conditions 3, 13, 24, 32, 181
cirrhosis 105-107
cirrhosis, ascites due to 107
cirrhosis due to qi and blood stagnation and stasis 105
cirrhosis of the liver 106

CONGEE LIST

197

A HANDBOOK OF MENSTRUAL DISEASES IN CHINESE MEDICINE by Bob Flaws ISBN 0-936185-82-1

A HANDBOOK of TCM PEDIA-TRICS by Bob Flaws, ISBN 0-936185-72-4

A HANDBOOK OF TCM UROLOGY & MALE SEXUAL DYSFUNCTION by Anna Lin, OMD, ISBN 0-936185-36-8

THE HEART & ESSENCE OF DAN-XI'S METHODS OF TREATMENT by Xu Dan-xi, trans. by Yang, ISBN 0-926185-49-X

THE HEART TRANSMISSION OF MEDICINE by Liu Yi-ren, trans. by Yang Shou-zhong ISBN 0-936185-83-X

HOW TO WRITE A TCM HERBAL FORMULA: A Logical Methodology for the Formulation & Administration of Chinese Herbal Medicine by Bob Flaws, ISBN 0-936185-49-X

IMPERIAL SECRETS OF HEALTH & LONGEVITY by Bob Flaws, ISBN 0-936185-51-1

KEEPING YOUR CHILD HEALTHY WITH CHINESE MEDICINE by Bob Flaws, ISBN 0-936185-71-6

THE LAKESIDE MASTER'S STUDY OF THE PULSE by Li Shi-zhen, trans. by Bob Flaws, ISBN 1-891845-01-2

Li Dong-yuan's TREATISE ON THE SPLEEN & STOMACH, *A Translation of the Pi Wei Lun* by Yang & Li, ISBN 0-936185-41-4

MASTER HUA'S CLASSIC OF THE CENTRAL VISCERA by Hua Tuo, ISBN 0-936185-43-0

MASTER TONG'S ACUPUNCTURE: by Miriam Lee 0-926185-37-6

THE MEDICAL I CHING: Oracle of the Healer Within by Miki Shima, OMD, ISBN 0-936185-38-4

MANAGING MENOPAUSE NATU-RALLY with Chinese Medicine by Honora Wolfe ISBN 0-936185-98-8

PAO ZHI: Introduction to Processing Chinese Medicinals to Enhance Their Therapeutic Effect, by Philippe Sionneau, ISBN 0-936185-62-1

PATH OF PREGNANCY, VOL. I, Gestational Disorders by Bob Flaws, ISBN 0-936185-39-2

PATH OF PREGNANCY, Vol. II, Postpartum Diseases by Bob Flaws. ISBN 0-936185-42-2

PRINCE WEN HUI'S COOK: Chinese Dietary Therapy by Bob Flaws & Honora Lee Wolfe, ISBN 0-912111-05-4, $12.95 (Published by Paradigm Press)

THE PULSE CLASSIC: A Translation of the *Mai Jing* by Wang Shu-he, trans. by Yang Shou-zhong ISBN 0-936185-75-9

SEVENTY ESSENTIAL TCM HERBAL FORMULAS by Bob Flaws, ISBN 0-936185-59-7

SHAOLIN SECRET FORMULAS for Treatment of External Injuries, by De Chan, ISBN 0-936185-08-2

STATEMENTS OF FACT IN TRADITIONAL CHINESE MEDICINE by Bob Flaws, ISBN 0-936185-52-X

STICKING TO THE POINT 1: A Rational Methodology for the Step by Step Formulation & Administration of an Acupuncture Treatment by Bob Flaws ISBN 0-936185-17-1

STICKING TO THE POINT 2: A Study of Acupuncture & Moxibustion Formulas and Strategies by Bob Flaws ISBN 0-936185-97-X

A STUDY OF DAOIST ACUPUNCTURE by Liu Zheng-cai ISBN 1-891845-08-X

TEACH YOURSELF TO READ MODERN MEDICAL CHINESE by Bob Flaws, ISBN 0-936185-99-6

THE SYSTEMATIC CLASSIC OF ACUPUNCTURE & MOXIBUSTION (*Jia Yi Jing*) by Huang-fu Mi, trans. by Yang Shou-zhong & Charles Chace, ISBN 0-936185-29-5

THE TAO OF HEALTHY EATING ACCORDING TO CHINESE MEDICINE by Bob Flaws, ISBN 0-936185-92-9

THE TREATMENT OF DISEASE IN TCM, Vol I: Diseases of the Head & Face Including Mental/Emotional Disorders by Philippe Sionneau & Lü Gang, ISBN 0-936185-69-4

THE TREATMENT OF DISEASE IN TCM, Vol. II: Diseases of the Eyes, Ears, Nose, & Throat by Sionneau & Lü, ISBN 0-936185-69-4

THE TREATMENT OF DISEASE, Vol. III: Diseases of the Mouth, Lips, Tongue, Teeth & Gums, by Sionneau & Lü, ISBN 0-936185-79-1

THE TREATMENT OF DISEASE, Vol IV: Diseases of the Neck, Shoulders, Back, & Limbs, by Philippe Sionneau & Lü Gang, ISBN 0-936185-89-9

THE TREATMENT OF DISEASE, Vol V: Diseases of the Chest & Abdomen, by Philippe Sionneau & Lü Gang, ISBN 1-891845-02-0

THE TREATMENT OF DISEASE, Vol VI: Diseases of the Urogential System & Proctology, by Philippe Sionneau & Lü Gang, ISBN 1-891845-05-5

THE TREATMENT OF DISEASE, Vol VII: General Symptoms by Philippe Sionneau & Lü Gang, ISBN 1-891845-14-4

THE TREATMENT OF EXTERNAL DISEASES WITH ACUPUNCTURE & MOXIBUSTION by Yan Cui-lan and Zhu Yun-long, ISBN 0-936185-80-5

160 ESSENTIAL CHINESE HERBAL PATENT MEDICINES by Bob Flaws ISBN 1-891945-12-8

630 QUESTIONS & ANSWERS ABOUT CHINESE HERBAL MEDICINE: A Workbook & Study Guide by Bob Flaws ISBN 1-891845-04-7

230 ESSENTIAL CHINESE MEDICINALS by Bob Flaws, ISBN 1-891845-03-9p